HEALTH AND HUMAN DEVELOPMENT

RANDOMIZED CLINICAL TRIALS AND PLACEBO: CAN YOU TRUST THE DRUGS ARE WORKING AND SAFE?

HEALTH AND HUMAN DEVELOPMENT

JOAV MERRICK - SERIES EDITOR –

NATIONAL INSTITUTE OF CHILD HEALTH
AND HUMAN DEVELOPMENT,
MINISTRY OF SOCIAL AFFAIRS, JERUSALEM

Adolescent Behavior Research: International Perspectives
Joav Merrick and Hatim A. Omar (Editors)
2007. ISBN: 1-60021-649-8

Complementary Medicine Systems: Comparison and Integration
Karl W. Kratky
2008. ISBN: 978-1-60456-475-4 (Hardcover)
2008. ISBN: 978-1-61122-433-7 (E-book)

Pain in Children and Youth
Patricia Schofield and Joav Merrick (Editors)
2008. ISBN: 978-1-60456-951-3

Challenges in Adolescent Health: An Australian Perspective
David Bennett, Susan Towns, Elizabeth Elliott and Joav Merrick (Editors)
2009. ISBN: 978-1-60741-616-6 (Hardcover)
2009. ISBN: 978-1-61668-240-8 (E-book)

Behavioral Pediatrics, 3rd Edition
Donald E. Greydanus, Dilip R. Patel, Helen D. Pratt and Joseph L. Calles, Jr. (Editors)
2009. ISBN: 978-1-60692-702-1 (Hardcover)
2009. ISBN: 978-1-60876-630-7 (E-book)

Health and Happiness from Meaningful Work: Research in Quality of Working Life
Søren Ventegodt and Joav Merrick (Editors)
2009. ISBN: 978-1-60692-820-2

Obesity and Adolescence: A Public Health Concern
Hatim A. Omar, Donald E. Greydanus, Dilip R. Patel and Joav Merrick (Editors)
2009. ISBN: 978-1-60456-821-9

Poverty and Children: A Public Health Concern
Alexis Lieberman and Joav Merrick (Editors)
2009. ISBN: 978-1-60741-140-6

Living on the Edge: The Mythical, Spiritual, and Philosophical Roots of Social Marginality
Joseph Goodbread
2009. ISBN: 978-1-60741-162-8

Alcohol-Related Cognitive Disorders: Research and Clinical Perspectives
Leo Sher, Isack Kandel and Joav Merrick (Editors)
2009. ISBN: 978-1-60741-730-9 (Hardcover)
2009. ISBN: 978-1-60876-623-9 (E-book)

Rural Child Health: International Aspects
Erica Bell and Joav Merrick (Editors)
2010. ISBN: 978-1-60876-357-3 (Hardcover)
2010. ISBN: 978-1-61324-005-2 (E-book)

Children and Pain
Patricia Schofield and Joav Merrick (Editors)
2009. ISBN: 978-1-60876-020-6 (Hardcover)
2009. ISBN: 978-1-61728-183-9 (E-book)

Conceptualizing Behavior in Health and Social Research: A Practical Guide to Data Analysis
Said Shahtahmasebi and Damon Berridge
2010. ISBN: 978-1-60876-383-2

Chance Action and Therapy: The Playful Way of Changing
Uri Wernik
2010. ISBN: 978-1-60876-393-1 (Hardcover)
2011. ISBN: 978-1-61122-987-5 (Softcover)
2011. ISBN: 978-1-61209-874-6 (E-book)

Adolescence and Chronic Illness. A Public Health Concern
Hatim Omar, Donald E. Greydanus, Dilip R. Patel and Joav Merrick (Editors)
2010. ISBN: 978-1-60876-628-4 (Hardcover)
2010. ISBN: 978-1-61761-482-8 (E-book)

Adolescence and Sports
Dilip R. Patel, Donald E. Greydanus, Hatim Omar and Joav Merrick (Editors)
2010. ISBN: 978-1-60876-702-1 (Hardcover)
2010. ISBN: 978-1-61761-483-5 (E-book)

International Aspects of Child Abuse and Neglect
Howard Dubowitz and Joav Merrick (Editors)
2010. ISBN: 978-1-60876-703-8 (Hardcover)
2010. ISBN: 978-1-61122-049-0 (Softcover)
2010. ISBN: 978-1-61122-403-0 (E-book)

Positive Youth Development: Evaluation and Future Directions in a Chinese Context
Daniel T.L. Shek, Hing Keung Ma and Joav Merrick (Editors)
2010. ISBN: 978-1-60876-830-1 (Hardcover)
2010. ISBN: 978-1-61668-376-4 (E-book)
2011. ISBN: 978-1-62100-175-1 (Softcover)

Positive Youth Development: Implementation of a Youth Program in a Chinese Context
Daniel T.L Shek, Hing Keung Ma and Joav Merrick (Editors)
2010. ISBN: 978-1-61668-230-9 (Hardcover)
2010. ISBN: 978-1-61209-091-7 (E-book)

Pediatric and Adolescent Sexuality and Gynecology: Principles for the Primary Care Clinician
Hatim A. Omar, Donald E. Greydanus, Artemis K. Tsitsika, Dilip R. Patel and Joav Merrick (Editors)
2010. ISBN: 978-1-60876-735-9

Understanding Eating Disorders: Integrating Culture, Psychology and Biology
Yael Latzer, Joav Merrick and Daniel Stein (Editors)
2010. ISBN: 978-1-61728-298-0 (Hardcover)
2011. ISBN: 978-1-61470-976-3 (Softcover)

Advanced Cancer Pain and Quality of Life
Edward Chow and Joav Merrick (Editors)
2010. ISBN: 978-1-61668-207-1 (Hardcover)
2010. ISBN: 978-1-61668-400-6 (E-book)

Bone and Brain Metastases: Advances in Research and Treatment
Arjun Sahgal, Edward Chow and Joav Merrick (Editors)
2010. ISBN: 978-1-61668-365-8 (Hardcover)
2010. ISBN: 978-1-61728-085-6 (E-book)

Environment, Mood Disorders and Suicide
Teodor T. Postolache and Joav Merrick (Editors)
2010. ISBN: 978-1-61668-505-8

Social and Cultural Psychiatry Experience from the Caribbean Region
Hari D. Maharajh and Joav Merrick (Editors)
2010. ISBN: 978-1-61668-506-5 (Hardcover)
2010. ISBN: 978-1-61728-088-7 (E-book)

Narratives and Meanings of Migration
Julia Mirsky
2010. ISBN: 978-1-61761-103-2 (Hardcover)
2010. ISBN: 978-1-61761-519-1 (E-book)

Self-Management and the Health Care Consumer
Peter William Harvey
2011. ISBN: 978-1-61761-796-6 (Hardcover)
2011. ISBN: 978-1-61122-214-2 (E-book)

Sexology from a Holistic Point of View
Soren Ventegodt and Joav Merrick
2011. ISBN: 978-1-61761-859-8 (Hardcover)
2011. ISBN: 978-1-61122-262-3 (E-book)

Principles of Holistic Psychiatry: A Textbook on Holistic Medicine for Mental Disorders
Soren Ventegodt and Joav Merrick
2011. ISBN: 978-1-61761-940-3 (Hardcover)
2011. ISBN: 978-1-61122-263-0 (E-book)

Clinical Aspects of Psychopharmacology in Childhood and Adolescence
Donald E. Greydanus, Joseph L. Calles, Jr., Dilip P. Patel, Ahsan Nazeer and Joav Merrick (Editors)
2011. ISBN: 978-1-61122-135-0 (Hardcover)
2011. ISBN: 978-1-61122-715-4 (E-book)

Climate Change and Rural Child Health
Erica Bell, Bastian M. Seidel and Joav Merrick (Editors)
2011. ISBN: 978-1-61122-640-9 (Hardcover)
2011. ISBN: 978-1-61209-014-6 (E-book)

Rural Medical Education: Practical Strategies
Erica Bell, Craig Zimitat and Joav Merrick (Editors)
2011. ISBN: 978-1-61122-649-2 (Hardcover)

Advances in Environmental Health Effects of Toxigenic Mold and Mycotoxins
Ebere Cyril Anyanwu
2011. ISBN: 978-1-60741-953-2

Child and Adolescent Health Yearbook 2009
Joav Merrick
2011. ISBN: 978-1-61668-913-1 (Hardcover)

Public Health Yearbook 2009
Joav Merrick
2011. ISBN: 978-1-61668-911-7 (Hardcover)

Child Health and Human Development Yearbook 2009
Joav Merrick
2011. ISBN: 978-1-61668-912-4 (Hardcover)

Alternative Medicine Yearbook 2009
Joav Merrick (Editor)
2011. ISBN: 978-1-61668-910-0 (Hardcover)

The Dance of Sleeping and Eating among Adolescents: Normal and Pathological Perspectives
Yael Latzer and Orna Tzischinsky (Editors)
2011. ISBN: 978-1-61209-710-7 (Hardcover)

Child and Adolescent Health Yearbook 2010
Joav Merrick (Editor)
2011. ISBN: 978-1-61209-788-6 (Hardcover)

Child Health and Human Development Yearbook 2010
Joav Merrick (Editor)
2011. ISBN: 978-1-61209-789-3

Public Health Yearbook 2010
Joav Merrick (Editor)
2011. ISBN: 978-1-61209-971-2

Living on the Edge: The Mythical, Spiritual, and Philosophical Roots of Social Marginality
Joseph Goodbread (Editor)
2011. ISBN: 978-1-60741-162-8 (Hardcover)
2011. ISBN: 978-1-61122-986-8 (Softcover)

Alternative Medicine Yearbook 2010
Joav Merrick (Editor)
2011. ISBN: 978-1-62100-132-4 (Hardcover)
2011. ISBN: 978-1-62100-210-9 (E-book)

The Astonishing Brain and Holistic Conciousness: Neuroscience and Vedanta Perspectives
Vinod D. Deshmukh
2011. ISBN: 978-1-61324-295-7 (Hardcover)

Translational Research for Primary Healthcare
Erica Bell and Joav Merrick (Editors)
2011. ISBN: 978-1-61324-647-4 (Hardcover)

Drug Abuse in Hong Kong: Development and Evaluation of a Prevention Program
Daniel T.L. Shek, Rachel C.F. Sun and Joav Merrick (Editors)
2011. ISBN: 978-1-61324-491-3 (Hardcover)

Human Development: Biology from a Holistic Point of View
Søren Ventegodt, Tyge Dahl Hermansen and Joav Merrick (Editors)
2011. ISBN: 978-1-61470-441-6 (Hardcover)
2011. ISBN: 978-1-61470-541-3 (E-book)

Our Search for Meaning in Life
Søren Ventegodt and Joav Merrick (Editors)
2011. ISBN: 978-1-61470-494-2 (Hardcover)
2011. ISBN: 978-1-61470-519-2 (E-book)

HEALTH AND HUMAN DEVELOPMENT

RANDOMIZED CLINICAL TRIALS AND PLACEBO: CAN YOU TRUST THE DRUGS ARE WORKING AND SAFE?

SØREN VENTEGODT
AND
JOAV MERRICK

Nova Science Publishers, Inc.
New York

Library of Congress Cataloging-in-Publication Data

Randomized clinical trials and placebo : can you trust the drugs are working and safe? / editors, Sxren Ventegodt, Joav Merrick.
p. ; cm. -- (Pharmacology-research, safety testing, and regulation series) (Public health in the 21st century series)
Includes bibliographical references and index.
ISBN 978-1-61470-067-8 (hardcover)
1. Clinical trials. 2. Placebos (Medicine) 3. Drugs--Toxicology. I. Ventegodt, Sxren. II. Merrick, Joav, 1950- III. Series: Pharmacology-research, safety testing, and regulation series. IV. Series: Public health in the 21st century series.
[DNLM: 1. Randomized Controlled Trials as Topic. 2. Drug Toxicity. 3. Placebos. 4. Treatment Outcome. QV 771]
R853.C55R36 2011
615'.10724--dc23

2011020025

Published by Nova Science Publishers, Inc. †New York

CONTENTS

PREFACE

Randomized clinical trials (RCT) have been accepted as the golden standard of testing making chemical medicine "evidence based". RCT is based on four assumptions: 1) The placebo effect is represented by a placebo pill, 2) it is possible to make a double-blind test with biologically active drugs, 3) beneficial and harmful effects of drugs are fairly measured in RCTs, and 4) an appropriate time frame for the test is used. We have found problems with these assumptions: 1) The placebo effect provided by close relationships to a physician is stronger than an inert pill, 2) double-blind tests cannot be made with biologically active drugs, as these leave an internal clue in the patient that destroys the blinding (active placebo), 3) lack of global outcome measures makes toxic effects invisible for the test and magnifies minor effects to make clinically insignificant positive effects look important, and 4) RCTs are used in such a brief time frame that side effects and harm are not properly detected. The four errors combine into a serious error: The RCT-procedure induces a strong bias in favor of any toxic drug tested. RCTs can turn drugs that are only toxic and not beneficial at all into products sold as useful chemical medicine. Many pharmaceutical drugs on the marked today are tested only with this flawed RTC-procedure and we recommend that these drugs be tested again using a rational method. If drugs are not more helpful than placebo we need to return to classic psychosocial holistic medicine.

INTRODUCTION

We live in a materialistic world. Materialism means that everybody believes in matter as the true essence of the world, not consciousness as our ancestors believed. We believe in natural science, in atoms and molecules as the fundamental parts of which the world consist. But in science we know that we cannot understand consciousness with molecular and physical–chemical models. The primary quality of consciousness is *oneness*: that everything is so closely connected that space and even time seems to disappear, when you go deep into the experience of reality.

Medicine comes in two versions, the old and the new: The consciousness-based and the biochemical, pharmaceutical medicine. The new medicine is the industrial medicine; huge pharmaceutical companies with tens or hundreds of thousands of employees and billions of EUROs and dollars in yearly turnover, which are driving the development of biomedicine forward.

There are strong common interests between governments and industry around medicine; to keep the society stable, productive and to keep the political power the population must be provided with medicine. As machines combined with information technology are highly productive and produced the work similar to 100 or 1,000 persons, we live in a rich world, where a few people can feed a large group. Therefore we observe that paradoxically population health is not necessary geared for high productivity; stability and political power to the people who wants to support industry is much more important. Modern biomedicine is playing an important role in the political play of power, securing citizens' satisfaction and political stability in the economically rich, modern society.

But when we look at population health in Denmark and other countries with socialized medicine, we can see that more than half of the population is chronically ill, and this in spite of intensive treatment with biomedical drugs. This makes many people wonder what is really happening in the modern world. Have we developed a system, where financial and political power is gained, while population health is lost? Have we developed a world where people are pampered with material wealth so much that they existentially are falling asleep in a kind of hypnosis of false satisfaction? Is the happiness and positivity of modern materialistic culture a total illusion, when it comes down to it? And does biomedicine play a major role in maintaining this illusion?

CAN WE TRUST THE RCT-TEST USED TO DOCUMENTS THE SAFETY AND EFFICACY OF MEDICINE?

What if the test procedure that is used by all pharmaceutical companies today to document medical drugs, shows the opposite of what it is intended to do? What if it turns everything upside-down, so poisons becomes medicine? What if there is so much money in selling this poisonous medicine that it displaces the old, established psychosocial medicine, and make everybody believe that the chemical medicine is the RIGHT medicine, even when it only harms the patients? And what if a large fraction of the billions of EUROs, pounds and dollars it earns every year is used to keep the people in the wrong understanding, with the intention to make even more money on this harmful medicine?

These were the questions that came to our minds when our international group of researchers first analyzed the randomised clinical trial (RCT), which today is the basis for almost all scientific trials of pharmaceutical drugs on human beings (1). We became interested in analyzing this procedure because of a significant and systematic difference between the test results from the pharmaceutical industry, and the independent groups of researchers' results, when they later critically analyzed the data from all the pharmaceutical trials.

Much too often did the pharmaceutical industry document that the drugs were efficient and relatively harmless, while the independent research documented – using exactly the same data – documented that the chemical medicine was both ineffective and dangerous.

In the beginning of our analysis we did not expect to find much. As we dug deeper into the material we found four errors, that did not look especially problematic, but as we took a closer look, we found that the four errors *combined* made the pattern that everything was turned upside-down. Poisonous drugs came automatically, as a consequents of the way the errors were combined, to look like efficient medicine, and harmful effects were hidden, when the drugs were tested using the standard RCT of the pharmaceutical industry.

The next question we had to ask was, if the pharmaceutical industry had did this on purpose, or if it just had happened through a coincidental development. We answered first this question for each of the four single errors, which all increased the probability of the pharmaceutical drugs looking good and being suitable for the market. Each of these four errors seemed to have been introduced by the researchers of the pharmaceutical companies as a conscious deception, and not by coincidence. But still, we could not be sure that the pharmaceutical industry had understood the combined effect, the fatal error, occurring from of the four minor errors.

If the pharmaceutical companies fully understood that the standard RCT makes poisons – biologically high active drugs with only harmful and no beneficial effects at all - look like efficient, harmless medicine, they would not use this method any more. Or would they?

In this book we show how the RCT-method makes it possible for the pharmaceutical industry to make billions of EUROs, pounds and dollars by selling poisons as medicine. We also document, based on established medical science, done by research groups independent of the industry, that large groups of pharmaceutical in use today, only are poisonous to the patients.

We have chosen to focus on the drugs that are used by the most ill patients: Cancer chemotherapy and the most used psychiatric drugs: the antidepressant and antipsychotic drugs. The studies we use as reference are large metaanalyses – studies that resume hundreds of scientific paper – made by established researchers at highly acknowledged research centers that are independent of the pharmaceutical industry.

These scientific studies are made by the most credible and trustworthy researchers, and of the very highest scientific quality – a quality superior by far to every single study made by the pharmaceutical industry used for documenting and marketing the drugs.

It is important for us to underline that we are believers in science, and that we are physicians with no negative attitude to medical drugs in general. We most certainly find that there are many drugs that can benefit the patients: Antibiotics like penicillin, painkillers like morphine, and hormones like insulin etc.

Our aim is not to reject all pharmaceutical drugs, but just to warn against the consequences that follow from the drugs not being properly scientifically tested, and the drugs not being used according to the highest and most valuable and trustworthy scientific knowledge, that exists about them.

In the end of the book we give our proposal for how to test chemical medicine, so we can be sure that the quality is good. For we believe that patients must have all the medicine that can help, independent of type. The good physician can use all methods and tools. But all these tools must be based on sound and trustworthy science.

On the other hand we find it highly problematic that convincing scientific documentation, of a quality so high that no researcher in the whole world has managed to find flaws in it, showing that the drugs really don't help but only harm the patients, not is leading to the withdrawal of the medical drugs. The products are still sold as if nothing has happened, and the medical industry defends its position by referring to their own documentation for the products. All this makes it extremely important to shed light into the problems that is regarding the RCT-method, which is the basis of the documentation. If the RCT is doubtful, the documentation is problematic. If the RCT is invalid, the documentation is useless.

We know from the statistics that every second Dane has a chronic disease, in spite of unlimited and free access to biomedical medical service (2). We know that almost every Dane frequently uses chemical medicine. Why don't the patients get well again then? Why don't the drugs cure them? It is not because the medical companies are not doing their best to make efficient and safe medicine, we are certain they are. Our answer is that it simply is impossible to cure chronic diseases simply with chemical medicine. It cannot be done.

That it should be possible is a sheer illusion created by the pharmaceutical industry by massive and constant marketing through decades. In our part of the world, the rich western world, a person gets ill sometimes because of lack of self insight and as a consequence a low quality of life, a bad job, unsatisfying relationships, and a poor and unhealthy lifestyle. The main cause of disease is psycho-social factors, and not bad genes. Not bugs. Not additives in the food. These traditional causes seem to contribute very little to our general unhappiness. You can't change psychosocial factors with a chemical pill, however magic the bullet may be presented.

To get well again you need self-insight and personal development. This is how it is today, and this is how it has been for millennia. The classical medicine is about the doctor helping his patient to gain self insight and develop his or her personal character. This is the original medicine that goes back to the father of medicine science, Hippocrates (3). The medicine that was here before Big Pharma took over.

If you have sufficient economical resources you can market and sell pills, effective or not, to all sick and suffering people of the world, if just you can make them and their doctor believe that the drugs are efficient. And if you do you make billions to you can afford more marketing. The primary condition to make people believe in pharmaceutical products is to make them appear *scientifically tested* and thus trustworthy.

How you exactly do this, even when the chemical substances used only are poisons, is the gigantic medico-industrial deception that we reveal to the world in the book.

May our work benefit all living beings.

Søren Ventegodt og Joav Merrick

Chapter 1

THE ERRORS AND DEFICIENCIES OF THE RANDOMIZED, CLINICAL TRIAL (RCT)

The concept of medicine covers a lot of subspecialties, many of which are of excellent value to modern man. It you get a bite by a tick and get Lyme disease, or if you are unlucky enough to get syphilis from unsafe sex, you will most definitely appreciate the penicillin cure, which will safe in the first example your life, and in the second your brain and your sanity. In the emergency room the lives of countless traffic victims are saved, and skilled surgeons are even able to saw arms, legs, fingers and toes back into place. If a dog molests a little girls face the likelihood is good that plastic surgeons will give her a new face.

If you feel bad you go to your general practitioner (GP) and if he is wise, he will behave like your best friend, take your hand and listen to everything you have to say until you feel so much better at heart, and encouraged to turn your attention back towards your troublesome reality and deal more constructively with all things. He will make you realize how powerful you are in creating your own life, wonderful or miserable according to your level of insight in yourself. In the night you will sleep better, and you head and neck will stop hurting. Such is the art of classical medicine.

We (SV) have spent a long period of time assisting the brilliant plastic surgeon Dr. Bolund at University Hospital of Copenhagen, and to see him give a newborn baby born with palate cleft a new palace and mouth was to watch one of the true miracles of life: The miracle of good medicine.

Let's start this book with an unconditional salutation to our amazing colleagues, the physicians, who every single day, out of the talent and good, compassionate hearts, help countless numbers of patients to survive, overcome even the most severe and troublesome of conditions, and improve their quality of life.

This book is not meant to demean medicine in general, but to celebrate it, and to show the whole world that has started to doubt in medicine that an old tradition of good, rock-solid medicine exists. We want it to be acknowledged and used widely and we want this treasure to be taken well care of by society.

Unfortunately good medicine is not what is happening in all the subspecialties of medicine today. We have found reason to believe that the treatments with chemical medicine for the most severe physical and mental disorders are not happening in good order, and this is most disturbing.

We have found reasons to believe that this area of medicine has been driven off track, because of strong commercial interests that is not serving the patient's best interests. This book is written in the intent to bring these disturbed areas of medicine back on the right track. We pray that this book will be read by everybody with the understanding that we want to help the world to grow and develop and its people to be healthy and happy.

We have not written this to harm the business or reputation of any specific pharmaceutical company or any specific pharmaceutical product. We do not believe any pharmaceutical company to be neither better nor worse than any other company. The pharmaceutical products mentioned in this book are neither worse nor better than so many other pharmaceutical products we could have chosen to focus on and criticize. What we are addressing is the problems of chemical medicine *per se*.

Please read this book in the understanding that we are extremely sad to learn that some parts of modern medicine does not help the patients as much as they are supposed to. We feel obliged as scientists to share our knowledge about this with the public. Obviously, nobody else will say this loud, in spite of so many medical experts knowing of these problems. We have heard that one cannot say these things publicly without getting into some kind of trouble. But we will not keep silent, because of the fear that is keeping so many other people from telling the truth. We simply have to tell you what is wrong with the chemical medicine and why this is so. We trust that you will appreciate our efforts.

TESTING OF CHEMICAL MEDICINE – FROM EXPERIMENTS ON ANIMALS EXPERIMENTS ON HUMAN BEINGS

Before a chemical medicine, a pharmaceutical, is tested on humans, it is tested on animals to examine it for serous toxic effects. The drugs that are used as medicine are biologically active substances, meaning that they almost always are poisonous drugs.

These drugs are so poisonous that the animals either die or suffer severe damage if the dose is high enough. In animal studies the researchers find the lethal dose: The dose that will kill the animal, in mg/kilo. They also estimate the minimal dose for non-lethal damage on lever, kidneys, the animals' embryos etc. A new drug uses thousands of test-animals as the results of the tests are *statistical*. After this the company looks for a specific, pharmacological effect that in theory might be helpful to a sick human being. As the animals normally are not sick this is very much about guessing.

When these numbers are known the next step is testing on humans in a pilot study, where it is established if the toxicological data from the animal studies can be referred to humans being. Will the test persons survive? Will they be harmed? On a rare occasion they die, sometimes they end up in hospitals, but most of the time they survive without any harm done. Many poor people are earning good money this way. The pilot tells if it is acceptable to upscale the experiment.

Finally the time has come to test the drug on real patients. The pharmaceutical industry has decided that the drug must pass a test where it is compared with an efficient, inert pill that normally contains chalk, sugar or the like. This is the famous *placebo pill* (from Latin: I please). The rationale of the placebo pill is that faith alone makes people better; if you believe that you are being treated this by itself will induce a positive treatment effect, i.e. an improvement in the patient's health. This is known as the *placebo effect.*

Medical Science and Medical Art - 60 Years Ago and Before That

Before 1950 the number of active medical drugs was very limited, but then penicillin became available for the physicians, and this caused a revolution in medical thinking. For the first time there was a highly efficient drug, curing horrible diseases like syphilis and did it almost without adverse effects. The logic of penicillin was also convincing: The fungi had made it as defense against bacteria, and we human being had eaten bread with fungi for millennia without any harm – anyone knows that a lot of green cheese is mold, and the cheese is still completely harmless.

So hurrah for penicillin! And hurrah for morphine, also a drug almost completely without adverse effects! And so forth. And so forth. And so forth. No not really. Most other drugs used as medicine today have adverse effects. These drugs are famous exceptions from the rule that all drugs are highly poisonous. They are only a little poisonous. But still many people die from penicillin allergy and overdose of morphine every year. They are not safer than that. The discovery of penicillin gave a new faith in the chemical medicine. Drugs that could cure patients could be made! And soon hundreds of pharmaceutical companies started to develop.

Before 1950 drugs were rarely used, simply because there were so few and the use of them were so limited. At that time medicine was psychosocial and focusing on the whole person, his or her life and thoughts, behaviour, relations, feelings, sexuality, work etc.

The treatment consisted of a combination of therapeutic talk and touch therapy – what is often today called mind-body medicine, or holistic medicine. A substantial fraction of the physicians used homeopathic remedies and character analysis, and other physicians, the allopathic doctors, used strong poisons for a short while, like Strychnine, inducing a strong active placebo effect (see below).

But the classical way of medical treatment was to intervene on mind and body at the same time, through deep existential conversations supporting the development of self insight, and therapeutic touch, helping the patient to get better in touch with the body and with feelings and sexuality and other aspects of the human character that needed to be developed.

This kind of holistic medical treatment had been practices all the way back in time to Hippocrates (3), also called the father of medical science. Hippocrates lived on the island Kos in old Greece, where he about 400 BC had his famous hospital, the ruins of which can still be inspected.

The purpose of the Hippocratic medicine was that the patient should "step into character", be the best version of him or herself and give his gift to the world (3) – the gift that is the essence of human life, meaning, coherence, quality of life, and love, which we have theorized about and called every ones "life mission" (the life mission theory) (4-14).

When a human being successes in developing self insight, and learns what it has to give to others, he or she becomes of value in all relationships, and thereby happy, and then again well. This is the fundamental idea behind the holistic medicine that our international group has been researching for almost two decades now, leading to about 30 research projects contributing to about 200 scientific papers (15-31), most of them listed in www.pubmed.gov and a dozen of books on quality of life, quality of working life and holistic medicine (32-45).

The man's character and his "essence" or purpose of life (life mission) contains, according to this line of thinking, his physical, mental, and spiritual talents. Disease is according to the holistic disease model (37-39,45-52) caused by insufficient self insight and self confidence making the person incapable of claiming his talent.

"Know thyself" has been the key to personal development and to healing every single disease and every other kind of human suffering since ancient time, and the role of the physician has, since the time of Hippocrates and presumably long before that been to support the patients self exploration and help him develop sufficient understanding of self and life to reenter reality as a talented, contributing, and valuable person.

Disease is caused by missing, wrong or with the Greeks imbalanced use of body, mind, spirit and heart (corresponding to the four elements earth, water, air and fire). At Hippocrates' time the physicians used the elements to help the patient experience these energies within themselves, which still today is an advanced treatment method well known from the science of CAM (holistic, complementary and alternative medicine) (52).

Sexuality has always been important for the holistic medicine, as the human sex is an important aspect of human character. The Hippocratic physicians considered a healthy sexuality essential for a healthy body and mind (53-58). The Greeks has a much more liberal and accepting attitude to human sexuality, as is seen in the art from that time, and the physician was also sexologist (3). Many of the sexology procedures in use by sexologists today are described in the well-preserved medical sources from 400-200 BCE with about 70 books on traditional holistic medicine collected in the Corpus Hippocraticum (3,59-63).

The writing of the medical books was essential for establishment of medicine as a science. The tradition of discussing every significant problem in the society of physicians to agree on the best solutions and to collect empirical data and logical principles on healing was the cornerstones of the emerging medical science.

Hippocrates called his science for "the art". *The art* was as much an art of living as it was an art of medicine. It was before all about the physician being an ethical person, coming from heart and good intent, and being of willing to serve others (3,64). For more than two thousand years the traditional holistic mind-body medicine was the medicine of Europe. A society of highly respected, noble men, the doctors serving emerged, men and later also women serving their communities at the best of their ability. Medicine became established in the consciousness of the people as a light in the dark, and as we shall see below, this psychosocial, person-oriented, and holistic medicine had the power to cure people from all kinds of illnesses, diseases, sexual, psychological and existential problems and to keep the population healthy. No wonder it was popular.

Biomedicine Takes Over

In 1948 the first trial using randomisation was done in Great Britain; it tested streptomycin for tuberculosis (67). The design soon became popular, and about 1960 many physicians considered the emerging, pharmacological, biochemical medicine more scientific and modern than the classical psychosocial medicine. Treating a patient with a chemical drug was so much easier than talking and touching for hours and years with patients. Naturally the new medicine had to be more efficient than the old one. When a chemical medicine was tested it was therefore important to compare the old, traditional treatment with the new. Unfortunately this was not so easy.

One of the major problems here were that the physicians attitude to the treatment in itself pushed the patient up towards health or down towards disease. If a physician was very positive towards the new chemical treatment and similarly negative towards the old, traditional treatment, the chemical treatment would work better. If on the other hand the old way was considered more safe and efficient, this would win over the new drug in the competition. The consciousness – the patients' conscious and unconscious mind – was the critical factor determining the outcome of the experiment. Because of this problem, the pharmaceutical industry needed a test method that could deal with this troublesome *placebo effect* (65), which was the basis of the classical medicine, but not the basis of the new chemical, more scientific medicin. At this time psychological factors were not considered a proper subject for science; it was only 20 years later, about 1980, that the science of psychology was accepted in most western countries.

The test method that was suggested and later became fully accepted as the scientific solution to the problem was, that the patient receiving the treatment, should be held in the dark regarding being in the treatment group or in the control group. The medicine should be tested *blind*. The physician giving the treatment should know neither which patient got the chemical treatment nor who got the placebo treatment. If he did this knowledge would introduce a bias making the result unreliable. Furthermore the two groups of patients should be comparable, which was why randomization was suggested. The test was therefore a *randomised double-blind trial against placebo* or for short *the randomized clinical trial (RCT)*(66).

The introduction of the RCT solved one problem but gave a more fundamental problem to the testing. If the patient receives a talk-touch therapy this is hard to hide. So the classical holistic treatment cannot be used in the RCT. As a placebo control was needed the pharmaceutical industry suggested that the placebo cure was represented by the placebo pill – a pill that looked exactly as the pill with the active drug. The industry argued that if the patient believed in the placebo pill, the placebo effect would still be there, so this was OK.

There were in the beginning many protests from physicians who felt that a companionate, deep-felt, honest talk about personal development, and a loving, caring supporting and accepting hand on the patient's body could not be well represented by a passive piece of chalk. By letting the new chemical medicine compete only with a passive placebo pill they got all too easy access to the market. In reality, biomedicine did not need to be better than the old psychosocial medicine at all, to be approved! Other doctors argued, from experiments that showed that up to 80% of the effect of morphine came from placebo, that the placebo pill was inducing a very strong placebo effect, and that it was the perfect control needed for testing the new pharmaceutical drugs.

As years went by the RCT method was first accepted by the medical journals and then by the physicians at the standard method for testing the chemical medicine on human beings. The protests died out. The commercial interests in the chemical medicine had by financial support and sponsorships a strong influence on the universities and the academic medicine, and the RCT method was also accepted here. Today the randomised clinical trial is the only method that is internationally accepted. You cannot test a drug any other way. So all new drugs are tested this way.

So every time the pharmaceutical industry tests a new drug on humans the patients will be divided by randomization, in a treatment and a control group. The treatment group will receive the active, almost always poisonous drug, and the control will receive an inert substance. The person that does the randomization is not the treating physician, so nobody knows who receive the active drugs and who don't. Or this is at least how it should be, according to the theoretical design. And then the patients is simply monitored for good and bad effects from the drug, and from the placebo, and finally compared statistically. This is how all drugs are tested today.

THE ASSUMPTIONS BEHIND TESTING MEDICAL DRUGS WITH THE RANDOMISED CLINICAL TRIAL

When the drugs are tested with the RTC-method the value of the drugs depends on this method. For a first look this method looks highly scientific. It looks simply as good as it gets in science. Designer drugs from expensive high tech chemical labs, experts and physicians in white coats, randomization, equality in the treatment regarding all psychological factors which hereby is scientifically eliminated, and finally scientific statistic calculations and publications of differences – advantages and disadvantages – the finest scientific journals. This is really the *brave new world*. A science freak gets goose bumps.

The problem that with the RTC the value of the drug becomes dependent of the scientific value of the RCT test. I think we all agree that the method for a first glance really look scientific and in any way proper and fair. But when you think about it the RTC method is build on some assumptions that must be fulfilled before the method is valid[1]:

1) The placebo pill can fairly represent the placebo cure – i.e. the traditional holistic physicians' psychosocial treatment using talk-touch therapy.
2) The patient can be tested double blind, without discovering if he or she got the active drug or not.
3) In the RCT test it is possible to measure the positive and negative effects (adverse effects and events) on the patients' health of both the active drug and of the placebo for a scientific evaluation and comparison.
4) The RCT-test must run long enough to show the effects and adverse effects. For the drugs that is used for years must the effects be measured for years and not only short term (3-6 month) and both short term and long term effect must be reported.
5) The researchers responsible for the RCT-tests must be competent, decent and honest people that do not cheat, manipulate, lye, or in other ways, consciously or unconsciously, introduce a *bias* to the experiment in favor of one side or the other. They most also tell the world openly about the test results, also when the results are not in the interest of themselves (or their employer).

BIAS IN PHARMACEUTICAL RESEARCH

These five criteria seem simple to meet. In practice we have often seen that the scientific testing which has been done by companies that made money dependent on the outcome of the study contained *bias* (67). Bias in research may be defined as "anything which tends to make a conclusion differ systematically from the truth" (67). Bias thus means that the survey is "colored" and contains elements that gives the experiment an increased probability to come out the way it is wanted and thus to favor the economy of the pharmaceutical company. In general we find it fair to say that the pharmaceutical industry has had difficulties with honoring the fifth criterion (67). A Danish doctoral thesis on "Bias in double blind trials" by the acknowledged Cochrane researcher Peter Gøtzshe found bias in practically all drug trials on painkillers (NSAID for rheumatoid arthritis), and concluded that "It is difficult to see the typical NSAID-trial as anything else but a commercial for the new drug." (67)

The simplest way to make a bias is simply to lie about what was found in the drug-test. An analysis of this problem in JAMA concluded that in 72% of 149 analytical studies published in the leading journals the conclusion (and the abstract) was not in accordance with the statistical results in the paper, but were significantly twisted in favor of the new drug (242). So in most of these drug-papers the pharmaceutical industry simply claimed the new drugs to be better than they actually were. In medical science the conclusion and the abstract is really what counts; so this kind of deception is very efficient. The content of the abstract is also what is communicated to the public through commercials few weeks after the approval of the drug.

Let's give an example of a little more tricky kind of bias. If you notice from in the pilot study that there is a tendency that a new drug works best for employed men about 20 years of age, the RCT could "by accident" have a lot of young active men. If the drug is intended for use in the older, retired population, this would be cheating, as the drug in reality hasn't been tested on this group.

There is a well-known problem of this type in the testing of influenza vaccine, which makes the information from the pharmaceutical industry less reliable, as pointed out by an English Cochrane Center Researcher, Tom Jefferson (68,69). We (SV) had the honor to meet Jefferson at a scientific conference two years ago, where he told us, that he received murder threats after his critiques in the Lancet and elsewhere (70); he was most surprised to learn that these evil threats came on emails sent directly from people in the pharmaceutical industry.

There are so many ways to cheat. You can calculate the statistics wrongly, you can reduce great scales to simple, dichotomous data and thus "accidentally" loose information of adverse effects making the drugs look better (done in 26% of the trials studied by Gøtzsche (67)), you can even use a lower dose when you test adverse effects than when you test the beneficial effects (called dose-response bias; sometimes the dose varied in the RCT-trials by a factor 10 without any explanation in the paper suggesting this kind of bias (67)). If other researchers have made studies that go against a new drug, the pharmaceutical companies can simply exclude these papers and use only the information that shows that the drugs works wonders and is not very toxic; and this is often done (67).

There are simply hundreds of different ways of cheating, and the pharmaceutical industry has been proven again and again to uses them all, as Gøtzsche showed in his thesis about the NSAID drugs. It was accepted by the medical faculty that these drugs had not been documented well, but these drugs continue to be in the shops of Denmark and the rest of the western world, and they are being used by millions of chronic pain patients every day. Millions of people who have been mislead to believe in the positive message on the label on the box, ensuring them that they will fell less pain when they buy and use the drugs. The sad thing is that they most probably don't.

Gøtzsche concluded that the hundreds of biases he found are most likely to be general problems with all the pharmaceutical industry's testing of drugs, and not only related to painkillers (67).

Today we know of plenty of cases where the pharmaceutical companies have not honored the fifth criterion (67,71). We all know about that – you cheat a little and are a little dishonest when this is in you interest. So we all understand this. To compensate for the weakness of human nature the national authorities of all developed countries control the pharmaceutical companies and have introduced plenty of procedures and rules in an attempt to avoid the cheating. Sometimes we don't, and this is not good for the patients, of course. But this is how life is. Shit happens.

Most physicians know of these problems, as anybody else do as they are often discussed in the media, and most physicians agree that the pharmaceutical industry could be more ethical but that we have to live with them as they are, if we want to have a medical industry at all. This book is therefore not about all the problems and sufferings that bias and lack of objectivity in the RCT-testing mean for the patients. It is about the fundamental problems with the method itself.

Are the Fundamental Assumptions Behind RCT Correct?

The focus of this book is on the problems regarding the first four criteria. As we shall see, there are so fundamental errors here that you cannot say the RCT-method is a scientific method. You cannot say that the RTC is useful for testing the chemical medicin. It cannot be used for documenting the pharmaceutical drugs.

At a time where the whole world seems to agree that the RCT method is OK, is acceptable, is great science, and that it is bad timing to criticize the method as all drugs now are based on it, we have found it invalid. It contains a series of errors that sum up to fatal error. It makes poison to medicine.

Imagine for a moment that the RTC-method isn't all right. That it is a method that Big Pharma has developed because it is in its economic interest, but that it is not in the patients' interest.

Imagine that it does not work. That it is not able to show if a chemical medicine has positive or negative effect on the patients' health. Imagine that the RCT-method make poisonous drugs without any specific pharmacological, helpful qualities at all appear as beneficial and almost harmless medicine.

Imagine for a moment that the RCT-method at its very roots is deceiving us. That it leads to the wrong conclusions. That it is a scoop for the pharmaceutical industry but completely without scientific justification. Imagine that the RCT method leads to lots and lots of different poisons being sold as medicine. That it causes that a huge fraction of people in the western world is poisoned without anybody noticing that. That people go to their doctor because you feel even worse after getting the drugs, because they are, and the doctor just tells them that nothing is wrong - and definitely not the drugs - and that they just have to live with it. And that thousands of patients even dye suddenly and unexplained from the adverse effects accumulating through time or even sometimes commit suicide because of severe chemically induced depression or low quality of life. If that really was the case, wouldn't it be important to find out?

After a thorough scientific investigation into the RCT-method, now published in a www.pubmed.gov listed journal, we believe this to be the case. We think the situation is worse than grave. As we as a single group of scientists cannot define reality or tell other people, scientists or not, what to think, we have written this book to take the subject to public debate.

In chapter two to four we will show the four errors that we have found with the RCT method. In chapter 6 and 7 we will discuss the impact on public health and public economy the blind acceptance of this flawed method has had. In chapter 8 will we document, using the metaanalysis made by solid researchers from research institutions independent of the pharmaceutical industry that large groups of pharmaceuticals are only harmful and have no beneficial effect at all on the patients. We have chosen the drugs used for cancer chemotherapy and for psychiatric treatment of depression and psychosis – the anti-depressive and anti-psychotic drugs – as our examples. In chapter 9 and 10 we will discuss the problematic aggressive marketing of the pharmaceutical industry, and the way biomedicine treats its enemies. We have already seen one example with Jefferson above. Chapter 11 contains our reflections on what it takes to improve the situation. In chapter 12 we give our suggestion for a rational test of chemical medicine in the future. And in chapter 13 we give a resume of this book for scientists, physicians and the academic reader. For further reading we refer to our scientific paper on the errors of the RCT method (1).

Chapter 2

PROBLEMS WITH THE PREMISES OF THE RCT: THE PLACEBO PILL HAS NO PLACEBO EFFECT AT ALL SO THE DRUGS WIN THE RACE. ALWAYS

THE PLACEBO PILL HAS NO PLACEBO EFFECT

In the randomised clinical trial (RCT) an active drug is tested against an inert placebo pill. This has been done for scientific reasons, to make double-blind testing against placebo possible. The placebo pill represent the power of consciousness to give the patient healing, i.e. the placebo cure, which only 60 years ago or so was the standard treatment given by the psychosocially oriented general practitioner, in the proud medical tradition of Hippocrates. In this tradition a combination of talk and touch therapy had worked wonders for millennia. Therefore, every physician those days knew and acknowledged the "power of the mind" - the healing power of the patients' consciousness, causing the placebo effect. It was in the end accepted that this placebo effect was represented by a placebo pill, in spite of the fact that holistic medicine was never practiced in the form of distributing placebo pills.

The assumption that the placebo pill could represent the placebo cure and had a strong placebo effect has recently been challenged. A new Cochrane metaanalyses has compared the placebo pill treatment with *no treatment* from a lot of three-armed studies having an active drug arm, a placebo arm and a *no treatment* arm, and concludes that there is no effect at all of the placebo pill in the RCTs (72). It was exactly as the silenced critiques had insisted on many years ago. The placebo pill had no effect at all.

So the assumption the pharmaceutical industry had that the RCT compared the active drug with placebo was totally wrong[1]. You may find this irrelevant today, but please reflect upon the fact that 2400 years of successful medical practice was exchanged by biomedicine, on this basis. The drugs have an easy game; there was no competition at all. The industry pretended to compare the active drugs with placebo but they did not. They compared with *no treatment*. So they succeeded in canceling the whole traditional, holistic medicine, with this trick. The pharmaceutical industry cannot just cancel 2400 years of successful medicine because you want to sell your drugs. That's really not acceptable. But it happened. And it happened because the pharmaceutical industry was so much stronger than the general practitioners, because it had allied itself with the universities and the academic establishment. The pharmaceutics industry did well. I attracted smart people, paid them very well, and got strong influence. It won the world. Today it owns the world. It dominates research at almost all universities in the western world. But it cheated. It never compared its healing power to the healing power of the classical psychosocial medicine. It cheated with a design that only pretended to do so. It was a fraud.

Obviously there are huge commercial interests in the chemical medicine. Everything you can put in a jar and sell in 80 million copies a day will make you very rich. This is the basic idea of the capitalistic society. But if the content in the jar does not work, and it has replaced an efficient medical treatment, then it is a disaster for the patients. If pharmaceutical medicine is less effective and more harmful that classical holistic medicine, then we don't need it after all. We need to use the old medicine that really works. Hands on, and empathic talks.

It is time to recall us that the physicians are there for the sake of the patients, not for the sake of the pharmaceutical companies. As physicians we can and shall not accept a shift from holistic, consciousness-based medicine to chemical medicine if we cannot be sure that this means better medicine for the patients. From the way the drugs are tested it is easy to understand that the likelihood that classical medicine is better is really high.

And to the argument that chemical medicine is more scientific than holistic medicine we want to say: It is not so. The psychosomatic medical theories of which there exists a large number of rather high complexity (46-52) are not less scientific than the biochemical medical theories. It is quite opposite. Holistic medical theories focus on the human being while chemical theories focus on molecules. Psychosocial medicine is focusing on experience, consciousness, quality of life, emotions, sense of coherence, sexuality, psychological and social factors. Chemical medicin is focusing on genes, molecules, intercellular signaling etc. The holistic theories are about the person and his or her disease or health issue. The chemical theories are about chemistry, of course. What has that to do with health? Very little! But the pharmaceutical industry insists that molecules and disease markers are relevant for health. But they are not. The majority of studies comparing hard and soft factors, chemical and psychological factors, in medicine find that the soft data is always “harder” than the hard data. The subjective health is always a better predictor for future survival and health that any objective medical factor, any blood test dimension, any hard chemical aspect (73-77).

It is not that we have anything against chemistry or natural science; quite opposite has this always caught out strong and dedicated interest. The first author can brag that he was the only student at med school in his year to get a straight A (13 on a scale from 0-13) in biochemistry, and we have even during the recent years made papers on the future development of the science of chemistry into a more complex, holistic quantum chemistry, that better could explain life (94).

We are not telling you this to brag but to let you know that we understand chemistry very well. We understand it so well that we have used the rules of chemistry to prove in a formal No-Go Theorem, together with the famous physicist professor Holger Bech Nielsen that biology – that biological form and order (morphogenesis) including the cellular dis-order that basically IS physical disease cannot be explained from chemistry, genes and DNA (91).

When the cells fine order is disturbed, so the cells don't know what to do anymore, the places they are in the body, we get arthritis, cancer, heart conditions etc. Chemistry cannot explain that. Biological order seems to come from another, more complex, source than DNA and chemistry, a source closely connected to our consciousness (17,87-108). This is why consciousness is so closely connected to health and disease, and chemical factors aren't.

But the goal of the pharmaceutical industry is never to research into these fundamental questions that always lead away from chemistry. The pharmaceutical companies are not interested in understanding life, biological order, health, quality of life and consciousness. They want to make money. That is per definition their aim. These companies are organs in a capitalistic society. They are after the money. Never never ever doubt that. Because this fact is the key to understanding the basic logic of the modern western world. That much we have learned being involved in medical research for several decades know.

In line with what we have told above, we know from all major, comparative studies that the self-assessed health is the hardest predictor of future health and survival that we have in medical science today (73-77). From this research we know, without much doubt as this tendency has been seen systematically in all major studies, that psychosocial factors are more important for health than biochemical factors. So this is the name of the game. Science has spoken. Improving quality of life and self-assessed health might be the direct and only way to better objective health. Quality of life is the best medicine as we recently concluded in another paper (111).

So we need to reconsider what happened the day everybody agreed that the holistic medicine and its placebo cures for almost everything could be replaced by an inert pill. That was stupid. That was dumb. Big Pharma got its way with the world, and chemical medicine replaced talking to the patient, caring, being there, showing concern and love, touching the sick body and comforting the suffering human being. All this was replaced by a chemical pill. Just because of money. Big Pharma won the world and all the patients of the world, and their physicians, lost.

This does not mean that there are no good drugs; some drugs obviously cure diseases and can be used as great medicine – penicillin for syphilis is a great example. But for most drugs things are not that clear, and a closer look will reveal the sad truth that the drugs are not very effective, but they are often harmful. Biologically active chemicals are often quite poisonous. And that is what is in the pharmaceutical pills, after all...

EFFICACY AND HARM OF BIOMEDICINE

As we said above the chemical medicine has almost never been tested against the classical, holistic medicine. Therefore we do not know the relative efficacy and harm of the two kinds of medicine from such studies. To compare the two medical systems we need to go another way, and look at the number of patients helped and harmed with the two very different types of medicine.

We have simple measures of efficacy and harm that allows us to do this comparison, called Number Needed to Treat to benefit (often just called Number Needed to Treat, or NNT), and Number Needed to treat to Harm (often just called Number Needed to Harm or NNH). This sounds complicated but is not. Number Needed to Treat is the number of patients you need to treat to help or cure one patient.

Let's take an example. You give penicillin to children with acute otitis media. You hope that it will prevent damage to the hearing, and that is one outcome. And you want the children to suffer less pain, that's another. How many children do you need treat for one to feel less pain? The answer is 15 (163), so NNT=15. How many patients do you need to treat to prevent loss of hearing? Infinitely many, as the drug does not do that (163) (NNT not defined as the treatment with penicillin does not have this outcome). How many kids are harmed, then? Well, we don't know. To know this number, you need to know how many children suffers from adverse effects from the penicillin itself, on short and long term (i.e. induced penicillin allergy from the treatment giving problems later), you need to know how many children are suffering from the administration of penicillin though injections, ill-tasting liquid medicine etc. And this information is not available. As a group of researchers we could of course found out. But we have chosen to focus on the severe physical and mental diseases in our research, and in this book. So we don't know. But in general there is one patient harmed (getting adverse effects) for three patients taking a pharmaceutical drug (NNH=3) (110).

In general the pharmaceutical industry has not been too happy with the concept of NNT and NNH numbers. It tries, for obvious reasons, to hide them. A few years ago UKs public media revealed to much surprise for its citizens that "The drug don't work"(79). The debate also appeared in the BMJ who let the whole world know, that in general the NNTs for pharmaceutical drugs are around 20: "NNTs under 5 are unusual, whereas NNTs over 20 are common." (79). This means that if you go to your doctor with a disease and gets a drug to treat it, you average likelihood to be helped by the drug is about 5%. You got 19 chances out of 20 that you stay ill.

But don't think that one in 20 patients is cured by the doctor, from these numbers. No no no. *One in 20* patients is improved on some measure that normally is a single symptom, or a disease marker, meaning a biochemical factor with some (often far) relation to a disease. So only one in 20 gets some help. In chapter 6 we shall show that in reality it is only one in a hundred or so, that is really cured by biomedicine. So what do you think? Is biomedicine efficient? Does it cure the patients?

If you want to know how efficient the drug you are taking for your health problem is, you need to find the NNT number. But this might be difficult know. In many countries, including Denmark, there has been a process going on of hiding the NNT and HHN numbers for the public. So if you go to a pharmacist in Denmark you cannot get this crucial piece of information. Your doctor does not have it either. You must write to the national board of health to get it. (So do that!) And this is how it is in many countries. You are not supposed to know that "The drugs don't work" (79). You are supposed to believe in chemical medicine, not for scientific reasons but for political and economical reasons. If you knew the NNT number you would hardly rely on this kind of medicine to get better, would you? You would not buy the drugs, would you? You would not go home and wait patiently to get better, would you? Of course you wouldn't. If you knew these things, you would this day find another treatment, and another kind of medicine that gives you better chances to get well again. So this cover-up is necessary for you continue to buy and use the chemical medicine. It's a capitalistic world indeed.

It has been amazing for us to watch the changes on national level towards biomedicine during the last 20 years in Denmark, with the removal of the NNT and NNH numbers from all the information material send yearly from the National Board of Health to all physicians and pharmacists in Denmark being an obvious and scary example. It has often been discussed if *Big Pharma* really exists. Is there an international union of pharmaceutical companies that coordinate the whole pharmaceutical industry's collective efforts to mould and shape the world, including the information that nations and states are giving to the physicians, pharmacists, and patients? Does the pharmaceutics industry really meet to discuss how to impact nations in the collective interest of the whole industry? What do you think? And how powerful would such a co-operation of the most powerful and influential companies internationally be in shaping the world? Chills down your spine?

Well, we have discussed this with a professor in business at an acknowledged Schools of Business, with focus on industrial politics and thinking, and he believed that the pharmaceutical companies to a large extent coordinate their efforts (228). *Big Pharma* seems to be a reality that we have to deal with. It's time for us all to wake up and understand how this world operates. The wakening is not pleasant.

In chapter 8 we will discuss the NNT and NNH numbers for the drugs used for the severely ill patients with cancer, depression and schizophrenia and similar psychotic mental illnesses. For these drugs we know, as we shall see, that the NNT numbers are 50 or more, while the NNH is about 1. Meaning that only one patient in 50 is helped (but not cured as these drugs do not cure diseases, as we shall see), while practically everybody is harmed by the drugs (81-86). It seems to be the rule that if you get as long as you get an infection or something similar, that the body in reality could cure by itself, the drugs has some effect (163), but when you catch a real serious disease, the drugs cannot help you any longer.

EFFICACY AND HARM OF HOLISTIC MEDICINE

The drugs can still block symptoms of disease, but biologically active, chemical medicine cannot improve the biological order of the organism, it cannot interact with us at the causal level of the disease. In our understanding this is only logical as disease is caused by disturbances in the organism on the level of the biological information, which is much closer to consciousness that to chemistry. It is therefore our consciousness is so important for our health, and that development of consciousness, self knowledge and understanding of life is central in the classical medical cures for physical and mental diseases[3]. All our research points in the direction of diseases simply being caused by disturbances in our consciousness (17,87-108).

The time has come to ask the same question as we did above regarding biomedicine: How efficient and harmful is the classical, psychosocial, holistic medicine? In a series of reviews we have found that about every second patient that went into treatment with a physical or mental disorder, or with a sexual, psychological or existential problem, were cured (NNT=2) (109-111). From a metaanalysis of the treatment of 16.000 patients of all different kinds treated in four different countries we found none of these patients harmed, except for a couple of patients who broke some minor bones during intensive mind-body therapy in Sweden (NNH=4000) (109). A review of all non-drug medicine showed only one severe adverse effect (brief reactive psychosis) and it happened for 64.000 patients (NNH=64.000) (122). And all such patients recovered after 14 days. Holistic medicine is not harmful at all, in accordance with Hippocrates ethics (3). Such results could never be obtained with drugs.

For a decade we have done clinical research in holistic medicine in the Research Clinic for Holistic Medicine and Sexology in Copenhagen. We have found the same NNTs and NNHs for our patients here, independent of their clinical condition, physical or mental disorder, existential or sexual health issues. After one year of treatment, and about 20 sessions in average, half the patients were cured (62,112-117). We found out, during these clinical experiments, where we used the classical Greek methods almost exactly as they were described in the Corpus Hippocraticum (62), that holistic medicine really is extremely efficient and not harmful at all.

After publication of these results, our research clinic in Copenhagen lost its funding. To express it mildly our biomedical colleagues working in the psychiatry were not too happy with our research in holistic medicine and spread an evil rumor – through the boulevard press - about sexual abuse in the clinic. This was later examined by the police that found nothing wrong with the clinic.

But the clinic is still today not funded, which happen to be the normal pattern for this kind of research (70). This is basically why we wrote this book. We want to tell the world what really is going on around medicine. And we want to raise money for more research in holistic medicine (we have since 1989 raised about 40 million DKR for the research, see Acknowledgments, Chapter 14), so we can continue to develop the efficient and harmless psychosocial medicine the millions of chronic patients in the world today need. We will not let Big Pharma win this battle.

It has been interesting for us that so many diseases, also the more severe, which are often completely out of therapeutic reach with the chemical medicine, often can be rather easily cured by holistic medicine, like mental illnesses (94-200) and a bad heart (coronary artery stenosis) (118,119). We have also learned that quality of life and maybe even survival can be improved for cancer patients (121). Chronic patients that seem to have no chance with biomedicine in general (110), as they stay chronic patients for life in spite of all drugs in the world, can very often be helped and cured with holistic medicine (NNT=2) (62,80,110,112-117,165,169). The placebo medicine is simply the most efficient and safe medicine there is (65). The pharmaceutical industry has never liked this fact much.

PROBLEMS WITH COMPARATIVE RESEARCH BIOMEDICINE VS. HOLISTIC MEDICINE

In principle the biomedical treatment and the holistic treatment can be compared simply by having a huge research unit, a research hospital (our dream to create) with two different departments, one for biomedicine and one for holistic medicine. When a patient is entering the door, he or she will be randomised to biomedicine or holistic medicine. If the patients could accept that, such a hospital could easily be built.

The problem is that the two different medical systems cannot really coexist in the same building. The cultures among physicians are so different that you cannot image it. The biomedical doctors want "processional distance" to the patients, while the holistic doctor wants "professional closeness". The biomedical doctors believe in mental analysis, exact diagnosis, chemical blood tests and advanced technology, while the holistic doctor believe in love and intimacy, human understanding and well supported self-exploration. Biomedical doctors believe in being experts, holistic doctors want to be the patient's best friend. Biomedical professionals are authoritarian, while the holistic medical expert tries his or her best to be the patients equal. This is so different that it hard to believe. They don't even use the same diagnoses as they understand the human being and its health problems in fundamentally different ways (46-52,78).

These two cultures cannot exist under one roof. As we learned when we had to separate the Quality-of-Life Research Center from the University Hospital of Copenhagen in 1994, for this to be owned and directed by ourselves thereafter. But still such the research hospital could be established, if it was lead by people like us who believe in both chemical and holistic medicine. Syphilis should not be talked away. Penicillin is an excellent choice. So we cannot do without the drugs. So this comparative research documenting which disease and health issues needs holistic medicine and which needs biomedicine should be done for all the diseases, where there could be doubt. Fortunately there is sufficient information now to establish this knowledge from metaanalyses, as we have already done for most diseases (62,80,110,112-117,165,169).

The problem with the comparative research is that most patients would not accept to be randomised. They often either believe in chemistry or they believe in holistic medicine. We see this in psychiatry, where many patients accept the treatment, but where as many patients avoid psychiatrists like the plaque. We see cancer patients who choose chemotherapy and cancer patients that travel the world to get a holistic cure. You cannot randomize these patients. They think. They know what they want. If they lose the lottery they will simply go somewhere else. Even in Denmark, where biomedicine is free and alternative medicine is paid out of the patient's own pocket we have a million of patient choosing to get alternative medicine each year (160).

It is true that many patients are confused and try both systems at the same time; unfortunately these patients often have a sad destiny. They get even more confused because of the loss of energy, ability to think and concentrate other adverse effects from the drugs, which often directly sedates them. Often cancer patients and psychiatric patients are so sedated and so exhausted from the adverse effects of the drugs they get that they cannot even think clearly enough to cooperate with a holistic medical treatment (81,134,136).

So holistic medicine is NOT complementary to biomedicine. That is a general misunderstanding. Holistic medicine is not complementary to biomedicine in the sense that patients can benefit from both treatments at the same time in some combination. This is only rarely the case. The two medical systems are only complementary in the sense that we need them both to cure as many diseases as possible.

To understand how different these two medical treatment systems are it is interesting to study the two educations that lead to the two different academic degrees there have been established in Europe. At the normal universities all over Europe you can get the masters degree in biomedicine (MD, MMedSci). At Interuniversity College, an EU-Leonardo da Vinci project collecting all knowledge on CAM and holistic medicine from 40 different research institutions from all over Europe, you can get the similar masters degree in CAM (EU-MSc-CAM).

We (SV) have both these degrees. We were most surprised to learn that practically not a single hour of the teachings, or one single page of the readings, where repeated in the two curricula. They were indeed complementary. When you compare the curricula you notice that they come from two different universes.

Biomedicine is maximum 50 years old, while the science of holistic medicine is at least 2400 years old. The first speaks about molecules, the latter about man.

To think that you can reduce a human being to medical chemistry is really a big mistake. We urgently need the understanding of the human being in medicine. The healing from the placebo effect happens in the close relationship between a patient and his or her doctor[131]. This relationship takes time and mutual efforts to build. It can never be replaced by a placebo pill.

It is true that we do not understand the placebo effect in its full depth yet. When Indian gurus like Sathya Sai Baba says "cancer cancelled" to a cancer patient who believe strongly in his divinity and the cancer then disappears completely, as often described by witnesses and patients (120), this remains a mystery, and most physicians today are skeptical because they don't attribute so much power to consciousness, and so much healing power to the placebo effect.

But sometimes this happens in randomised clinical trials done at the best universities, by well respected physicians and researchers, as it did in 1989 when David Spiegel published his finding in the Lancet of radical improvement in quality of life and survival time when female patients with metastatic breast cancer improved their quality of life under his therapeutic leadership. He used methods from the classical holistic medicine, and he seemingly got the same results at the classical holistic physicians used to get (121). Several of the patients in the treatment group had spontaneous remission of their cancer and lived more than 10 years. None of the patients in the control lived more than five years. The miracle had happened at Stanford University also.

Conclusion

The pharmaceutical industry has managed to cancel 2,400 years of traditional medical practice, being successful ever since Hippocrates, by the assumption that the holistic placebo cure was well represented in the pharmaceutical trials by the placebo pill. But this assumption has not been proven wrong. The placebo pill has no placebo effect, as the placebo effect primarily lies in the relation between the patient and his or her physician.

During the last 30 years there has been more and more research in holistic medicine, done by physicians who felt that psychosocial medicine still had something to offer its patients. At a large number of research centers worldwide has it been proven that almost any disease and health problem, including sexual, existential and psychological, and including the most severe diseases as a bad heart, cancer and schizophrenia, can be helped and often cured by the placebo cure of the classical holistic medicine.

Recent reviews and metaanalyses by our group has documented that one in two of the patients could be cured with holistic medicine (NNT=2); the same number for biomedical drugs are about 20 (NNT=20). While almost all biomedical drugs have adverse effects (NNH=3) there are almost never seen side effects from holistic medicine and non drug CAM (NNH=64.000). Furthermore many more clinical conditions could be helped by holistic medicine, as the cure is basically about getting self-insight. From this we can conclude that holistic medicine is about 10 times as efficient and about 20.000 times as less harmful than the drugs (the chemical medicin).

Most interestingly this is not new to the medical society. Many times these arguments for CAM - that it is highly efficient also with chronic patients, and completely without harm - has been presented in estimated scientific journals as the Lancet (as we saw above), BMJ (British Medical Journal) and JAMA (Journal of the American Medical Organization) (123-128).

At the same time we have lots of huge metaanalyses, as we shall see for some of the most serious physical and mental illnesses that clearly documents that the drugs does not help the patients, but only destroys their quality of life and shortens their life (see Chapter 8).

Something is obviously wrong here. The pharmaceutical industry has succeeded in reducing classical holistic medicine to a placebo pill, a piece of chalk. The drugs have competed with nothing and had won the competition. That was smartly done. But it was cheating. And the whole world was deceived for a moment. But now we know, and the question is what we shall do about it. How we shall get the traditional holistic Hippocratic medicine that cures most patients without harming any, back.

Millions of chronically ill patients need it badly.

Chapter 3

PASSIVE OR ACTIVE PLACEBO?

The next serious problem for the randomised, clinical trial (RCT) seems to be of little significance for a first glance, but the deeper you look the worse it gets. This problem changes the sign of the test result from minus to plus: The more poisonous a drug is, the better it look in the RCT-test. The more harmful it really is, the more beneficial it will be documented to be in the RCT test.

The problem is that the placebo effect is strongly boosted by the feeling of getting an active drug. The stronger the drug is felt in the body, the more will the patient feel the "medicine" and be willing to change believes on life, health and destiny. I positive and constructive philosophy of mind encourage self-exploration and use of talents, and in this change of personality and lifestyle, the patient will get better. So even a strong poison can help a patient who received this as part of a medical treatment. The feeling of the "medicine" meets the patients' needs for signs of medical help and improvement.

A poisonous drug will impact body and mind, thus breaking the blinding of the RCT test as patients on an active drug can feel drug in their system, while patients on the passive placebo can't. That the patients get this placebo boost from sensing that they are on an active drug is well known in medical science as *active placebo* (66,132). Experts in medical test methods seem to agree on this phenomenon's existence and significance (66,132).

A poison can almost always be felt in the body or mind at some level, more or less unconscious but still significant for boosting the placebo, when it is used as medicine. And such use has a long tradition as we shall see.

THE HISTORY OF MEDICAL USE OF ACTIVE PLACEBO IN EUROPE

About year 1900 the classic holistic physicians had company of two other kinds of doctors, the homeopathic and the allopathic doctors. The homeopathic doctors were still working in the tradition of Hippocrates with the primary goal of improving and developing the human character of the patient, but Christian Friedrich Samuel Hahnemann (1755-1843) modified the classical treatment to include a treatment with a placebo drug, the homeopathic medicine. Hahnemann's "Organon" is still the authoritarian source for millions of physicians worldwide, and today about 10% of all medical treatments are homeopathic.

The allopathic doctors used the active placebo from poisons for treatment. The physician used a short, intensive treatment with a strong poison, i.e. strychnine, and the patient were sent deeply into a healing crisis, that turned every understanding of life, self and reality upside down. The poisons were really used as mind-expanders. The feeling that the medicine worked and that they just have to let go and trust in the doctor and the healing often helped, and the allopathic physicians were strong in their belief. Allopathic medicine was the *right* medicine.

The problem was of course that too many patients died or were harmed from the treatments, creating a strong interest in using new drugs. Many drug companies started to develop better drugs, and over the years, allopathic medicine developed into the biomedicine of today.

The allopathic doctors were good. They understood the active placebo effect, and they knew of course that the drugs they used for medicine were extremely poisonous. The developed a treatment still of “hit and run”, the patient had an almost lethal dose of poison for a short period of time, and then there was a complete withdrawal of the drug again, allowing the patient to recover before serious harm was done to the body. Sometimes the treatment was prolonged, and the patient went into a phase dominated by the symptoms from the poisoning. An active treatment cure thus had two phases, an active placebo phase with a healing crisis, and a toxic phase. The art of the allopathic doctors was to stop the game while it still was good, taking the patient of the poisonous medicine before he or she entered the toxic phase.

Historically seen the use of pharmaceutical drugs is rather new; the Hippocratic doctors used medical herbs but only outside the body. They had the firm believe that drugs were harmful and that medicine before everything else should be safe: Primum non nocere, first do no harm (3). This was the essence of the famous Hippocratic ethics. So they could not use drugs. And the Hippocratic physicians did not do that for more than two millennia. And the Hippocratic medicine was the dominating medicine in Europe since year 400 B.C. It was *non-drug* medicine. But then came the industrial age.

THE HISTORY OF MEDICAL USE OF ACTIVE PLACEBO IN PRE-MODERN CULTURES

Active placebo has been used in most pre-modern cultures as medicine, presumably also in Greece before Hippocrates and the western culture’s medicine. Shamans, medicine men, witches and druids have used plants and hallucinogenic mushrooms for thousands of years on the medical systems of all continents. The Native Americans from the north used magic mushrooms containing the hallucinogenic drug psilocybin, medical cactus like Peyote and San Pedro contained mescaline, and hallucinatory plants like Datura Stramoni, "Devils Apple", that contained scopolamine.

In the south the tribes used the hallucinogenic plants of the jungle two make the LSD-like Ayahuasca. In ancient Egypt they used the LSD-like Ergot alkaloids from mushrooms on wheat, and in Africa the sangomas extracted the drug Ibogain from plants. In central Europe the used with the Datura family (scopolamine), Mandrake (Mandragora Oficinarium) and Henbane containing hyoscyamine. In Northern Europe the same healer and shamans used the Fly Agaric mushroom (Amanita Muscaria) containing the hallucinogenic drug muscimol.

An analysis of the drugs used for shamanistic healing shows that the pre-modern cultures have had intimate knowledge of psychopharmacology and toxicology, as they have managed to find the least poisonous drugs that could give active placebo, the hallucinatory drugs, and use these as medicine. The only way they could have done that was by taking the drugs and in their own bodies learning about their effects.

It is amazing to learn that almost all pre-modern cultures have managed to identify the hallucinatory drugs available from natural sources that have the least adverse effects (171-174). Of all the drugs mentioned above only hyoscyamine and scopolamine are poisonous and harmful to the body. In spite of the horrible, public image of the hallucinatory drugs most of them are not poisonous at all. You cannot die from taking an overdose, your body cannot be harmed, and if you are not severely, mentally ill there is no likelihood at all for you committing suicide on the drugs (122).

Many western therapists, psychologists and psychiatrists have these active placebo drugs since 1960, where the drugs became known in the west, and researchers using these drugs often report large benefits for the patients whose whole personality and philosophy of life are dramatically transformed under the impact of the active placebo effect (175-178). Today millions of young people worldwide treat themselves with NMDA (Ecstasy), a drug with a moderate hallucinogenic effect, for solving and overcome their emotional, social and sexual problems.

In spite of the possibility of using active placebo the Greek Hippocratic physicians chose not to. The reason for this is simple: They did not need the drugs to induce the healing. Instead they used the combination of talk therapy, often talking about the most difficult and intimate things including sexuality, and therapeutic touch. The skilled holistic physician can, by using the natural, basic tools of talk and touch, impact the patient stronger than any drug, and induce a stronger placebo effect. Love and compassion are the unsurpassed tools for healing. No drugs can compete with love. No medicine is stronger than self-awareness and insight into the Self.

The Hippocratic doctors emphasized love, care and the patients intimate sharing of everything with the doctor, and therefore these physicians didn't need to use drugs at all. And this is how the holistic physician still works today: Helping the patient to explore him or herself and to heal all old wounds on body, mind and soul, using natural methods. This way the holistic physician cures most of his patients, even the most chronic and difficult, without the use of any drugs at all (80,111,122,135,165,169). But it takes a while, often a year or more to cure a patient.

The only thing you have to admit the pre-modern shamans and medicine men using the active placebo drugs is that they are damn cost-effective. While a holistic doctors is working for years on his patients, a good medicine who masters his magic tools can – at least according to the literature - often make the existential healing happen in only one day using his extremely dramatic and intensive, healing rituals (165,169,171-177).

By the way the hallucinogenic drugs have been banned in most of the western world. Why? Well the politicians do not like them. Why is that? Because everybody knows from the media how dangerous they are. Says who? Well, the psychiatrists that knows these things from scientific investigations, of course.

But this is not so. Recently the director of the psychopharmacological department of Kings College were fired because he publicly had said that LSD and similar drugs were less dangerous than alcohol and tobacco, after having documenting this in the Lancet (241). He said that because that is what we know about these drugs from science – it is quite well known, actually. Then, as he is supposed to be UKs leading expert on these matters, why was he fired? Because the politicians did not like what he said. Why? Well, you see, the politicians seem to be under influence by some leading psychiatrists that do not like these drugs. And why is that?

... well, for no scientific reason, obviously. But presumably because of a general fear of expanded consciousness and then these drugs cannot be patented, and sold as pills you take three times a day. It is quite the opposite way round: the active placebo effect of these drugs is so strong that you can use them to cure yourself. The placebo effect is so strong that you don't even need a doctor. And you only need to take these drugs a few times in your life, as this is enough to make the change happen, if you get a good look into yourself, so that you understand the real cause of you health problems.

These drugs are understandably a threat to commercial, chemical medicine, and basically also to the stability of the materialistic society. They threaten the authoritarian order of society at its root. Many critiques like the famous author and philosopher Aldous Huxley (1894-1963) stated often publicly that the psychedelic drugs could help people develop their consciousness and understanding of themselves – the drugs open people's eyes and make them believe more in themselves, they help people assume responsibility for own life and health, and often they make people rebel against the materialistic values of capitalism. This might very well be true and also the reason why they were banned. Huxley died even on LSD, believing this made his death easier.

This said, we do not advocate the use of hallucinogenic drugs as we do not believe them to be necessary in medicine at all. They might be useful to some groups of patients, but they are really not doing anything to a patient that a skilled holistic physician cannot do better.

The Use of Active Placebo in Modern Medicine

When we understand the dynamics of active placebo, we can also understand what happens if we put a poison, a drug that only has adverse effects i.e. nausea, and no specific pharmaceutical beneficial effects at all, through the standard RCT. If you compare a poison to passive placebo, the inert placebo pill (chalk), the poison has the ACTIVE placebo effect and wins the race. If you measure over a long period of time so the toxic effects dominate, this will not be so of course, but if you measure only short term, any poison will win. And we shall see below, practically all pharmaceutical drugs are only tested in the short term for adverse effects. So any poisonous drug will always win the race.

We know what you think now: It cannot be so simple to expose the cheating of Big Pharma. Trust us: It is. The problem of active placebo in the RCT test has of course been known for years, and in the beginning the pharmaceutical industry tested their drugs against active placebo. It was quite a disappointment for the new pharmaceutical test-drugs did not come out any better than just poison. But then, the modern type RTC was invented, using only passive placebo, and then the results were better. Therefore the pharmaceutical industry fought a fierce struggle to get the RCT accepted, and they did.

But still today, when we compare the drug, as we recently have seen in a Cochrane metaanalysis of the antidepressant drugs, these drugs are not significantly better efficient than the active placebo effect of just poisons (132). The pharmaceutical companies use the RCT test to document that these drugs help one in three of the depressed patients! And they do of course because of the active placebo effect that really is a powerful helper in the short (very short) run. But the anti-depressive pills do NOT contain drugs with any specific antidepressant effect, as the pharmaceutical industry has the nerve to claim. They contain poisons. And every researcher in the pharmaceutical companies working on antidepressant with these drugs knows that.

The problem here is not that the patients are being helped, because they are, in the short term. They believe they are helped and so they are. The problem is that the patients do not know what is going on, and that they keep taking poisons for years, and this is definitely not good for them. The drugs are only tested short term, as we shall discuss below, so neither the physicians nor their patients knows about the long term toxic effects; so they presume there is none and continue to take the poisonous drugs for years. In a time where everybody is so consumed with organic food, sustainable living etc. this deception is outrageous. If patients know, they would not take these drugs. They would not buy these drugs. They would not make the pharmaceutical industry rich. Which is why the patients are kept in the dark, of course.

What about the other drugs used in psychiatry, the antidepressant drugs? Well, as we shall see in Chapter 8 they are not better. Another Cochrane metaanalysis concluded recently that these drugs do not improve the patients mental health (the outcome is called "mental state") (133). In spite of being dozens on the market and the pharmaceutical industry again and again claiming that the drugs help the mentally ill patients, this is not so. Antipsychotic drugs, independent of type, are also only poisonous (133). And they are even more poisonous than the antidepressant drugs that are rather strong poisons. The antipsychotic drugs actually seem to increase mortality (209). This will be documented in chapter 8.

In general, all drugs that are tested and found to be effective drugs in the pharmaceutical company's standard RCT-test must be suspected to be either poisonous or strongly poisonous. In spite of what the label on the glass tells you.

We call this deception, because we know that the pharmaceutical industry knows that this is a fraud. This is cheating. The pharmaceutical companies do not tell anybody, because they want to make money. But independent researchers document in indisputable research of the highest quality, that they are selling poisons as medicine. We don't find that ethical. At all. We think it's a scandal.

The problem with using active placebo as medicine is not so much that it does not help the patients, because it does. The Native American medicine men and the shamans of the world would not be held in so high regards if they did not contribute and improve peoples' health. They do of course. The church had its fight against the withes in medieval Europe who were burned in millions because the witches were held in high regard and threatened the church because they knew how to heal with herbs and the priests did not. Spiritual healing might work but is not very efficient these days (122), while the active placebo drugs used by the witches really kicked ass (122). Active placebo works.

The problem is that the drugs sold by the pharmaceutical industry have a rather modest active placebo effect, just strong enough to for the drugs to pass the RCT, but not so strong that the patients gets hallucinations etc, so even if you take them for long the active placebo from them is not doing much for you, and at the same time they are very poisonous (81,134-136). All the chemical medicine does give a small active placebo effect in combination with a rather severe toxic effect. This means that the pharmaceutical drugs can pass the RCT-test and get a fine label as active medicine to the container for patients and doctors to read, but statistically it cannot improve the patients' health at all, as we have seen in Denmark (2).

Instead of an efficient placebo cure, as the one induced by a Hippocratic non-drug treatment with talk-touch therapy – or a shamanistic treatment with drugs that also would work as in modern drug-assisted psychotherapy with NMDA – the modern medicine goes in between.

Its pharmaceutical drugs look helpful and the principles in use are also real medical principles, but still the commercial medicine has no value to its patients. The patients are not cured, but have to use the symptom blocking drugs for life as chronic patients, and this is in reality what makes the pharmaceutical companies earn billions.

The patients are tuned into chronic patients and the stockholder into billionaires.

In countries like Denmark, were we are having free access to biomedicine (182), one in two is a chronic patient now, and the health of the population is constantly deteriorating[2]. The pharmaceutical industry has made a strong alliance with the state and has in reality taken over the power of medicine and led the whole western world into a horribly destructive path.

Much of the medicine used in psychiatry is so sedating that it is impossible for the patients to learn and develop as a person; the most serious side effect of antipsychotic medicine seems to be a loss of general ability - including sexual ability, social ability, working ability, and studying ability – caused by toxic effects of the drugs. The patients end up in institutions instead of being cured.

These general, "global" adverse effects are systematically avoided as outcomes in the RCTs when the psychiatric drugs are tested, in spite of their obvious necessity. As we shall see in the next chapter, the outcome measures of the RCT constitute another highly problematic area of the RCT.

The Significance of Active Placebo for the Scientific Value of RCT

The occurrence of active placebo effect in the RCT means that you cannot test a biologically active drug blindly, so in reality the RCT is not blind. It is double-blind in the beginning of the experiment, but as soon as the drug starts to know, the patient who received the active drug and not the inert placebo pill will know for sure that he or she is in the treatment group. The whole purpose of the scientific test design is destroyed by this. The RCT, randomised to be scientific, only looks like a scientific test from the outside. From the inside is it just active placebo. The patients know. The RCT cheats. RCT is not a scientific test, because it is not scientific at all, it is just a scamp. It's a make-believe to fool the world.

For us the real problem about the fake RCT is that the medical companies know – and have known ever since the beginning of drug testing – that the active placebo effect runs the show. They know that this golden, scientific test turns poisons into precious, marketable medicine, falsely labeled with the invalid results from the testing. And they don't seem to care as long the drugs makes money.

Why don't the national health authorities ask for better documentation? Well, maybe the people employed here is not that smart. Or maybe they are under some kind of political or economical pressure. We doubt that they are directly on the pay role of the pharmaceutical companies but we are sure that they would not be employed for long if they demanded a testing of all drugs against active placebo. Because then the drugs would not be approved and the pharmaceutical companies would have to close their factories. And this will not happen because the pharmaceutical industry is powerful enough to prevent it from happening – as it has been for many years. But it is time for national authorities to wake up and starting to demand that the pharmaceutical companies test the drugs with a rational method, not RCT.

To the patients of the world we want to say: Don't take these drugs anymore. They are not good for you. You have been fooled. And so have your doctor. Big Pharma has fooled us all. Stop buying its products, until they have been better tested. Stop believing the text on the labels of the tubes and scientifically looking medical glasses and bottles and fancy looking containers for drugs. Do stop it today, for your own good.

THE POLITICAL SITUATION AROUND MEDICINE

Who can do something about this sad situation? What about the medical associations of the world? Don't they have power to request decent documentation of the medical products? Not really, because as the society is constructed, the state or nation has this obligation. So the medical associations have to request this from the national health organs, which then must refer to a law, and all the laws about drugs have been under severely influence from the medicinal industry's lobby known to be one of the strongest and most influential in the world.

So now we come to you. You have the power to vote good honest men into the government, who are strong enough to take the fight with the pharmaceutical industry; ten minutes after the minister of health starts such an endeavor he will be on the front page of today's newspapers with some biomedical doctors, normally a group of psychiatrists with close links to the pharmaceutical industry, claiming that he neglect the patients needs, causes the patients to die from lack of treatment, or commit suicide because they cannot control themselves without the drugs etc. This always makes good stories and the people almost always believe the doctors in the media standing in their white coats and not the politicians, who what to "steel the patients' life-saving medicine just to safe society for a few bugs".

In the end the true power of medicine is in your hand. You need to understand what medicine is really about – and it is not much about chemistry but almost always about consciousness (29,65), as we have seen above – and you need to vote for people who are bright and comes from good intent, and you need to stop buying and taking poisonous drugs.

We also think the medical journals have an obligation to present medical issues fair, balanced, honest and scientific. We have the joy of serving as editors on several scientific journals, and we are reviewers on a dozen or so other scientific journals. We need the medical journals to be brave, and to also bring the analysis that is not popular with the industry. We have sadly learned that even the most acknowledged medical journals have been rejecting what we think is fine research in medicine that just is not in the interests of the pharmaceutical industry. And we must request that all medical journals in the future are far more critical when it comes to publishing drug studies based on RCTs.

The problem of the classical holistic medicine is that it fits poorly into modern industrial society. First you cannot make much money on a medical philosophy that believes that "the doctor is the tool" (129). Then modern man is so afraid of feelings, emotions and touch, that most of us would prefer a pill to a holistic medical treatment, if it was efficient in curing us and harmless. But for most diseases it isn't.

Then there is the question of competition. Marketing power is connected to commercial power and industrial success. Holistic physicians using their hands to cure patients will never be able to match Big Pharma. But the media could involve themselves in critical analysis of medicine, and if the truth were brought to the people about the relative efficacy of holistic medicin and biomedicine, and the relative harm done, this could easily balance the industrial commercials. Because people are not stupid.

To change from biomedicine to holistic medicine take a lot of courage for a physician who has been trained in biomedicine. It is easy to write prescriptions, its fast money and little work. Talking with patients is more difficult but also more interesting. Touching to heal is completely different from touching to examine. The moves might be the same, but the intention comes from a different place. Examination comes from the mind; healing touch comes from the heart. Most medical doctors have become so mental that it's a hard fight to get back into their bodies to feel and embrace their patients. But it can be done.

A physician who is trained in biochemistry might live a whole life without realizing that the only power found in the drugs is active placebo. He or she will often believe strongly in chemistry as the way to helping patients, because that was what was though at university. But the curriculum of the medical schools has been strongly influenced by politics and business. Wisdom was not where it came from, but from political reality.

WHAT CAN WE DO AS RESEARCHERS?

The first thing we can do as medical researchers is to investigate thoroughly into the questions of *what* cures the patients and *why* efficient medicine actually works. For the last 20 years we have been doing that. Now we know.

The next thing we must do is to tell our colleagues about it. We have during the last decades written over 200 scientific papers on quality of life and holistic health and published these in more than 20 different scientific journals. Today we have more than 130 papers on holistic medicine and quality of life listed in www.pubmed.gov. Now they know.

The third thing to do for us is to tell the public about it. Since 1991 we have appeared about 2,000 times in national media, mostly in Denmark. Now people in Denmark know.

We have done a lot already. But Denmark is small.

The reaction to our work has been very positive from thousands of Danish people. And it has been as negative from our biomedical colleagues. Some physicians, often psychiatrists, have called the Foundations supporting us telling lies to deprive our projects of funding. They have succeeded but again and again have we found new sources for funding, today being the most successful fundraisers in the area of holistic medicine in Scandinavia at all times.

As we got more famous, our biomedical colleagues have told horrible lies to the public about patients who we made crazy and abused violently and sexually. At some occasion the police were even asked by the National Board of Health (Sundhedsstyrelsen) to investigate these horrible accusations, but the police found nothing wrong with the clinic at all and that all evil rumors were not true.

We do not want to complain, because it has been a good life, and first of all we have chosen this life as researchers in psychosocial and holistic medicine ourselves. We knew from the beginning that we would swim against the current and that it would not be easy. But the game is getting tougher, we are stepping it up, and so are our opponents. To win now we need your support to take it to the next level.

What we want to do before we die is to stop poisons from being sold as medicine, and the whole world and everybody in it to be chemically polluted.

We want medicine to be once again an honorable endeavor, where the doctor cares about his patients and is efficient and able to cure his them without harming anybody. We want the physicians to be trained to deliver this kind of medicine to the world. We want holistic medicine to return to the university curriculums at all med schools of the world.

We need medical science to develop fast. We need the world to learn the ways of holistic medicine, not the old, traditional ways because these are somewhat old-fashioned, but modern ways to practice the same medicine, with a contemporary feel, but with a much deeper scientific understanding of the process of healing than the old Hippocratic physicians had. And therefore even more efficient.

But in the end it's the same medicine. We need to keep what is good and true about medicine. We have had this unique, precious eternal diamond of wisdom that has been polished in our culture for several thousands of years to shine at its brightest. But suddenly we have by accident dropped it in the sand of the pleasant beach of modern financial wealth; we have lost it out of sight for a moment, but it is not lost for good. We will keep on looking for it till we find it again, this precious gem of medicine. Because we can't live without it.

Chapter 4

MEASURING THE EFFECT OF DRUGS IN RTC. SHALL DOCUMENTATION BE BASED ON DISEASE MARKERS, LOCAL SYMPTOMS, OR GLOBAL DIMENSIONS OF SELF-RATED HEALTH, QUALITY OF LIFE, AND ABILITY?

How the outcomes are measured in the RCT, is very important for the result of the test[237]. If you look at the patients' quality of life, in an overall global measure, normally using a questionnaire, you can see the total impact of the drug – or any other treatment - on the patients' general wellbeing, including his or her self-assessed health and ability. If a drug does something good for a patient, it will increase the patient's global quality of life, and if it harms the patient, the quality of life will go down.

This is simple to measure in an RCT; it takes less than five minutes for the patient to fill it in before and after the treatment. The smart thing about using such a global measure is that the positive and the negative effects of the drug are measured in the same time. In this way a patient and his/her physician can know it the drug in general is useful. This of course is no guarantee that it will help the patient, as not every patient is helped by a treatment. We leaned above that it takes a certain number of patients, the Number Needed to Treat (NNT) to help one patient, and in the same way it takes a certain number of patients, the NNH, to give the patients a specific harm.

If one counts all the beneficial effects and ads their likelihood, one can calculate the total likelihood to get better (NNT_{total}), and if one counts all adverse effects and reactions to the drug one can calculate the total likelihood to get harmed (NNH_{total}). Normally there will be only one beneficial effect of a drug and 20 different adverse effects, so the NNT_{total} will be equal to the NNT but the NNH_{total} is often much larger than the individual NNHs. Because of this the NNT_{total} and NNH_{total} are never calculated by the pharmaceutical industry. Quite the opposite is happening: The list of adverse effects gets more and more specific as time goes by, making the NNH-numbers go up and up and up. As the NNH number used for the drugs are normally the lowest, signifying the highest risk, the drugs NNHs goes up and up and up, making everybody believe that the new drugs are safer than the old drugs.

We tested if this was so adding all the NNHs of the antipsychotic drugs to the NNH_{total} for each type of drugs, and found that the drugs are as harmful as the old ones, in spite of the

NNH seemingly going up (81); a large Cochrane metaanalysis of the antipsychotic drugs has recently reached the same conclusion (133).

At the same time the pharmaceutical industry is developing more and more specific outcome measures for the positive effects of the drugs, now totally leaving the patient and his/her disease to focus on biochemical "diseases markers", factors that are only statistically connected to a diseases. Again the NNT-numbers goes up, while the clinical significance of the drug is going down (237).

In this way, the result of the RCT-test is to a large extent a product of the chosen outcome measures. During the last 50 years we have seen a very sad development in these measures away from the patient and what is relevant for him/her, towards chemistry and extremely local aspects of health and disease.

The pharmaceutical industry has every years "improved" its outcome measures, and the people controlling the industry in national health organs and scientific ethical committees have been fast asleep not noticing this developing and its sad consequences for the patients: That less and less efficient and presumably also more and more poisonous drugs have been approved as "evidence-based" valuable medicine.

Another way of cheating is the documentation of small effects, which in reality is to modes for the patient to benefit. If you take the outcome "cured" this outcome is obviously of value to the patient; if you take the outcome 50% improved, this is still nice, but not a cure of course; the patient has still his/her disease but just less symptoms. But what about "10% improved" and "20% improved", as if often used in the (dichotomized) psychiatric studies?

Imagine this outcome combined with an NNT of 3: How interesting is it for a patient to know that one patient in five is 10% improved? What is my likelihood to be cured, then? Well, presumably, the NNT for "20% improvement" is about NNT=6, "50% improvement" is about NNT=20, and "cured" is like NNT=100.

We understand why the pharmaceutical industry would go for a small improvement in the outcome measure; it gives so much better NNTs. The doctor will tell you that "this drugs help one in three of patients, scientifically documented". Well, this may or may not be true (depending on the general validity of the RCT test), but what is the clinical value of it? And what about the adverse effects? What if the total likelihood of getting an adverse effect (NNH_{total}) is 1 or 2? Then it might be of less value that the drug helps one in three. More patients will be harm than helped, so the drug has limited therapeutic value.

If one in hundred is cured and everybody is harmed by this drug, is it worth a try? But if one in three is helped and one in five is harmed, this might be OK, right? Recall that for most drugs the NNT is about 20 (79) and NNH=3 (80). If a drug gets very fine, low NNT and great high NNH numbers you should check the outcome measures carefully. They are probably manipulated as described above.

Another bias in the RCT caused by the outcome measures it the RCT-tests failure to detect minor harms (like dizziness and loss of energy), and global harms (like compromised social ability). Only the adverse effects of the checklist will be registered. This does not mean that there aren't other adverse effects. It just means that the pharmaceutical company got away with only documenting these.

In the game of spotting bias and errors in the RCT one should always recall that the drug company wants to make money. It is not there for the patients, in spite of its claims. It is there for the stockholders. It wants to maximize its profit. And the better it can make the new drugs look, the more money it can make. The way the RCT-outcome is measured in practically every single drug trial is a clear example of this. But neither the patient nor the physician reads the protocols of the RCTs. They are long and very boring. They just read the product information. So they don't know what is really going on. Both of them trust the national control organs to take care of criticizing the protocols. But nobody is really making any demands about fair and clinically relevant outcome measures. Because all these organs are filled with strong believers in biochemistry. A skeptic sitting there and demanding better industrial testing would not survive for long.

THE OUTCOME SMOKE SCREEN – ANTIPSYCHOTIC DRUGS

Often more than one beneficial outcome in included in the RCT, especially if the outcome of main interest is difficult to establish. In the mental disorders, the patient's *mental health* is of major interest. As it is difficult to measure health itself, the scientists measure the patient's *mental state*, which is the outcome of major interest. Basically this measure is about how fearful, hallucinated etc, the patient is. It is closely related to the patient's quality of life. Most unfortunately this outcome is never improved by the antipsychotic drugs (81,133).

There is another outcome called behaviour (hallucinatory behaviour), which is really the patient behaving like crazy. This outcome is often improved, because the patients are pacified by the drugs that are strongly sedating (81,133). Nobody is really impressed by this; if you hid them with a hammer or gave them destructive brain surgery this would give almost the same result. But then, there is a measure called "Relapse". This sounds nice. It really is only "relapse of hallucinatory behaviour", not relapse of the bad mental state as this is never improved by the drugs. But "relapse" sounds like something that is good to avoid, doesn't it? Even if this only means that the patients are stoned by the toxic effect of the drugs. But is does not stop there. A smart mixture of mental state and behavior is called "global impression". This sounds relevant, doesn't it? If the *global impression* is improved, it must mean that the patient is somewhat better? Again, the words cheat. "Global impression" only means something like the mean value of the measured value of the outcome "mental state" and "hallucinatory behaviour".

As the improvement of "mental state" is always zero in these trials, the NNT of the outcome "global impression" is half the improvement of "behaviour". But it is so much nicer! So this outcome measure is often used. It makes everybody believe that the antipsychotic drugs improve the patients' general state of being. Even the physicians are fooled to believe this. And you need to read thick scientific (complicated!) papers to find out, and who has time for that?

And what do you think the pharmaceutical companies writes on the label of the drugs container? That the antipsychotic drugs do not improve the patient's mental state? No, they do not. It's a business. Would the patients take the drugs if that was obvious that the drugs didn't help them? It's important to fool people to keep the business running.

THE HISTORICAL DEVELOPMENT OF HOW THE POSITIVE AND NEGATIVE EFFECTS OF DRUGS ARE MEASURED IN THE RCTS

During the decades the testing of drugs has been more and more focused on specific symptoms or biological details and less holistic. It has lost its original focus on the patients' experience of being ill or well, documented by self-assessed health measured, quality of life ratings and measures of general ability. It has been less oriented around the patient, around the disease itself and its reasons, and more and more focused on specific organs or lately even on biochemical "disease markers", also called "surrogate outcomes" (237) which are concrete biochemical findings (like a high calcium carbonate contents in bones or a low cholesterol level in blood) that in other studies have been found to correlate statistically with the occurrence of a disease, or a symptom of a disease.

In this movement away from the human being and deeper and deeper into the biochemistry of man, it has been still easier for the pharmaceutical companies to document their drugs (237), and in the same time the drugs are doing still less for the whole patient and his or her global state. It is true that weak bones are correlated with an increased number of fractures, but drugs that increase the calcium carbonate in a patients bones have paradoxically been seen to correlate with more patients' bone fractures, not less, and if you lower the blood cholesterol level of a healthy person (which is often done) this patient has an increased mortality[237]. So surrogate outcome measures of often strongly misleading. But if you see this from the pharmaceutical industry's perspective, it is so much easier to make a drug that does something on a biochemical level than to actually help the patients and improve their health. During the last 50 years we have learned that the latter is virtually impossible.

30 years ago pharmaceutical companies normally tested the effect of their drugs using questionnaire to the patients and their physicians. These questionnaires contained measures for positive and negative effects of the drug treatment. To test the outcome of the drug intervention the patients of the RCT were then, as they are today, separated in two groups by random: The experimental group and the control group. All patients are measured before and after treatment (and often many times during treatment also).

The positive measures were some global health measures like self-rated wellbeing and quality of life, subjective physical or mental health, and often also some measures of self-related ability, like social ability, sexual ability, working ability, and studying ability. The questionnaire also included more local measures of the single symptoms of the disease or clinical condition which the drugs was intended to help on.

The negative effects were organized the same way, so the patients rated the overall experience of having side effects, and also the specific adverse effects of the drugs.

The questionnaires were fine tools for such an evaluation of the drugs. In a questionnaire it is possible in a short time to collect a huge amount of extremely valuable data about the patient and the treatment, and this cost almost no money.

Actually the data coming from self-evaluation (self-rating/ self-assessment) of health are the most valuable data we have today about health (73-77). The self-rated health is the best known predictor of future health and of survival (73-77). If you feel good, if you feel well, you will probably stay healthy and live for a long time. If you feel bad, you will probably get sick and dye rather soon. That's the statistic.

Close to the experience of health is the experience of quality of life (28,243). This connection is so strong that if you know the patient's quality of life, you can predict his or her health, even if you don't know the persons lifestyle[243]. The subjective dimensions of life have in a long series of scientific studies been shown to be what is important to health. So do yourself a favor and stay happy. If you are not, improve your quality of life, for this is the best medicine (21,138,139).

What was generally learned through these studies were, that the global measures of self-rated health, quality of life and general performance, showing the total effect of the drug on the patients mental and/physical health, quality of life, and abilities, were rarely improved by drugs, actually almost never, while the more local symptoms involving only one organ or one much more narrow aspect of life, often were blocked.

To improve the measures, the pharmaceutical industry has removed the global questionnaires in most drug trials, and replaced them with biochemical tests and questionnaires about specific things, like hundreds of different very specific side effects.

The most problematic thing about the pharmaceutical industry's documentation of the harmful, adverse effects (the side effects) has been the splitting of these effects in a large number of concrete specific effects; by having split the harmful effects in a number of specific effects each of these effects are statistically more rare than if these effects were grouped together, making the NNH-numbers go up and up. This is very smart, but it is a trick and what really interests the patient is: how often will I get an adverse effect from this drug. But this information is not provided anymore by the drug companies. So nobody knows.

We have added all these individually rare effects up to a total likelihood of having an adverse effect for the antipsychotic drugs (called "NNH total"), and we have found that every single patient is likely to have adverse effects from these drugs ($NNH_{total}=1$) - independently of drug type - in spite of NNH often reported as being 2, 3 or 5 dependent of the drug (81). So by this smart ways of counting, the high likelihood of harmful effects from the drugs is well hidden by the pharmaceutical industry.

So just by "improving" the outcome measures, the pharmaceutical industry has managed to make the drugs look much better and much less harmful.

CANCER CHEMOTHERAPY

If a cancer drug use for chemotherapy is tested using the outcome "cured" there is rarely any improvement. If you look at the outcome survival time, this seems to be improved for a few types of cancers (lung cancer, see chapter 8). If you look at the outcome quality of life, we know that the outcome is normally negative (see chapter 8). If we look at the size and number of tumors, chemotherapy will much often seem to work as the tumor shrinks immediately, when exposed to extremely strong cytotoxic drugs. If you look at the number of cancer cells in the blood carrying the chemotherapy around in the body, it is most likely that any strong cytotoxic drug will "improve" that. The narrower you look, the larger is the benefit.

As you can imagine the commercial game of the pharmaceutical industry is almost never to document cure of improved health or quality of life, as the drugs does not have such an effect, but only local effects that allows the drugs to be approves and aggressively market as highly efficient new drugs with less adverse effects than the old ones. Why do we call it deception? Because it is. You buy and use a pharmaceutical drug because you think it is good for you, but it is not. You have been fooled. But not only that. The doctor treating you has been fooled also. Because he is trained to believe in drugs, and the crucial information he needs to identify this drug as a poison is kept away from him. The pharmaceutical industry simply does not provide the data as they do not make them. The RCT does not examine them.

The silliest thing is that there are national committees on all countries controlling and approving the research protocols. But who is sitting there? You guessed right, biomedical physicians, also trained to believe in drugs. They will not demand global measures, NNT numbers for the outcome "cured", total counts of NNH etc. They are happy just to see a tumor shrink. Because this is in most cases as good as it gets with biomedicine for cancer these days.

So we have seen the sad degeneration of the positive RCT outcomes during the last 50 years, going from questionnaires measuring global dimensions of health and happiness, to biological samples, chemical and physical tests, advanced high-tech scans and now often disease markers not even directly related to the disease. At the same time the negative RCT outcomes have been more and more specific, making the NNH-numbers artificially go up and up. Making everybody believe that the new drugs were better and less harmful than the old drugs, which has not been the case for the types of drugs our group of researchers have investigated (81,86).

Once again the pharmaceutical industry has won the game. With the new top-tuned industrial outcome measures thousands of new drugs can be fabricated and approved, almost without any connection to something clinically practical and valuable for the patients, and without giving the patients and their physicians a fair impression of the toxicity of the drugs.

TESTING THE DRUGS: VIAGRA AS EXAMPLE

Let us give an example, analyzed in greater details elsewhere (238). Male erectile dysfunction may be improved by Viagra, as documented in the RTC studies (229). We know that erectile dysfunction almost always is caused by emotional problems in the relationship to the partner (240). We also know that the quality of the relationship and the level of sexual satisfaction are closely related to the quality of life. While Viagra might improve male sexual satisfaction, it might be correlated with increased sexual problem in the female partner (238,239), probably indication that the total sum of happiness in the relationship is not increased by Viagra; the quality of the relationship is not improved, and the man's quality of life is therefore not much improved in spite of his ability go get an erection. If you measure the outcome as penile hardness you can document a positive effect; if you measure male sexual satisfaction this becomes more difficult, and if you measure the patients global quality of life in dimensions like self-assessed quality of life (with questionnaires like QOL1,QOL5, QOL10, SWEQOL etc) it is most likely not to be improved at all; as the emotional distance that is the basic cause of the problem, and as this distance is thought to increase from the use of a mechanical mean of support like Viagra, the long term consequence of the use is more likely to be a lower quality of life. As quality of life is closely related to general health though the self-assessed men and physical health, strong predictors of health taken down as quality of life goes down, the total long term effect of Viagra might very well be loss of health. Add to this adverse effects of the drug Sildenafil to at least one in five (NNH=5) (228).

To market the drug the pharmaceutical company measures many different aspects, including the sexual satisfaction of the women. IF the company got lucky the patients' females partners statistically would experience an improved sexual satisfaction, and this would be great for the marketing: Take it for the sake of your women! She needs it. Obviously the study did not show that, as the pharmaceutical company withheld the data on the partner. So from this we can extrapolate the effect on quality of life of Viagra to be negative and the local effect on the hardness to be positive. A long term study is likely to come out worse than a short-term study. In this way, by adjusting focus of outcome and making it narrow, and reducing time to a minimum etc. the company can document a positive effect of Viagra that might not be there at all.

The pharmaceutical treatment of impotency helps as we saw technically one in three (NNT=3) (228) and harm, according to a metaanalysis, one in five (NNH=5). NNH_{total} is not known but is likely to be significantly higher than 5. The patient is not cured with the drug; he needs it for every single intercourse. The treatment is only symptomatic, which is typical when you treat with drugs.

In comparison the holistic treatment of male erective dysfunction, that was introduced by Masters and Johnson, addressed the true cause of the problem, the emotional dysfunction, and cured 2 out of three men (NNT=1) and had no side effects at all (240). As emotional healing is part of the sexual healing, both physical and mental health is improved in holistic sexology (114).

So while it seems easy to use, highly practical, and convenient for a man to take a drug for male erective dysfunction, in the long run it does not cure the patient, it gives many patients adverse effects because it is poisonous, it helps technically one man in three but seem to harm the relationship and quality of life, and in the long run even health.

If the drugs were decently tested the user would know that from the information on the package. Now the patient gets a positive impression of Viagra, and he can even brag to his friends and proudly tell that he has got access to this scientific wonder. When he chooses Viagra instead of holistic sexological therapy, he chooses a path that statistically leads him downwards towards hell, unhappiness, disease and emotional loneliness. He could have chosen a more difficult way, self exploration and personal development, and climbed the mountain of human happiness and health instead. This is the problem with the pharmaceutical medicine: So many patients are cheated to believe the drugs are good for them and in this way deprived the psychosocial cure that in reality is the only known real and lasting solution to their problem.

THE QUALITY OF LIFE QUESTIONNAIRES

The saddest thing is that measuring self-assessed health, quality of life, and ability is easy as it takes the patients about 5 minutes to fill in a five or ten question questionnaire (QOL5, QOL10) (138,139). Other fine questionnaires might take a little longer (138-141). Such questionnaires are inexpensive, and extremely informative. We know from a huge body of research that the information gathered in this way is unsurpassed by any other information you can collect about the patient, to predict his or her future health and survival (73-77).

There are a number of not-so-bad questionnaires that could be used to illuminate more specific aspects of the patients' health; some are made by researchers in the pharmaceutical industry 30, 40 and 50 years ago, other by good clinicians wanting to see good results of their treatments. The problem with these questionnaires is that they are not based on any theory; they are simply collections of all the questions the doctor felt was relevant that day (ad hoc collections of questions) (40,41,147).

The best questionnaires are developed by holistic researchers focusing on the whole person in the global dimension quality of (138-140), sense of coherence (SOC) (155,156), self-assessed physical and/or mental health (138-140), and social, sexual and working/studying ability (139). We are proud to say that our group has developed a number of these questionnaires. We have also used much effort and time analyzing the existing questionnaires to improve them (i.e. Antonovsky's SOC questionnaire (230-235)).

The reason for *not* including such essential questionnaires as RCT outcomes is of course that the pharmaceutical industry *never* would include outcome measures that documented that the drugs did not help the patients. Why shoot yourself in the foot? And what do you think, is the outcome "the patient died spontaneously", "the patient committed suicide" normally or not normally included in the drug trials?

And the people who has the power to demand that such measures are included are either fast asleep or on the pharmaceutical companies pay role one way or the other (including doing sponsored research, or making a living from selling the drugs as biomedical physicians). Big Pharma is everywhere.

Other more resent questionnaires are highly problematic; they are seemingly developed by the WHO like the global mental health questionnaire WHOQL5. It does not measure global quality of life (global QOL) as it says but only depression. It has been developed by people employed by the pharmaceutical industry obviously to argue that more people in the world should take antidepressant drugs. The fact that WHO for years has been dominated by Big Pharma and now seem to serve mostly as the a brilliant platform for industrial marketing of new drugs to the whole world, the new swine flu vaccine being an example, makes us very sad. Really sad. WHO was created to help the world. Now it helps the pharmaceutical industry to sell poison and destroy it.

CONSEQUENCES OF BAD TESTING OF THE ADVERSE EFFECTS

We know that all biologically active drugs are toxic. Even the drugs that are identical with the drugs that are naturally present in the body, like insulin. Just the way they are administered to the body leads to adverse effects. Toxic drugs often compromised the general level of life energy and alertness. In young people normally used for the testing of pharmaceutical drugs this effect is not dramatic. But old people can get really low and dizzy because of the poisoning, especially when they are given many drugs at the same time, which is quite normal.

When we as you doctors worked in the hospital we often saw old people that could not function in their own home anymore, but as soon the about 10 different drugs (one for each major organ system in the body) they used were withdrawn, they came back and 14 days later, when they were "de-toxed" they could think, talk, read and orient themselves again, and return to their home. It is easy for GPs to ad a drug, but always risky to take it away. Nobody will blame you for treating the patient, but neglect (not giving the drugs if they are needed) would be severely punished by the national authorities. The first author of this book has for the last four years been under investigation by the Danish medical authorities for not giving drugs (with the medical license temporarily suspended). In Denmark not giving drugs as a GP, but using holistic medicine instead is a crime severe enough to make you lose your license...

Big Pharma is not that different to Orwell's famous Big Brother. Mind control and control of all physicians' behaviour. Fear and severe punishments for not obeying the command: "You must push drugs. You must push drugs. You most push drugs."

As with the positive effects of the drugs, the negative, adverse effects can be measured globally using exact the same global measures of health and quality of life. But this is never done. Often the patient is monitored with a questionnaire listing all the concrete presumed adverse effects. But there are often more side effects that the ones the pharmaceutical industry happens to expect.

We all recall the problematic drug Vioxx, the pain killer taken by 80 million patients that most experts now believe gave thousands of patients acute myocardiac infarction and stroke; most health professionals will also know that the company behind it in 2008 paid the victims or their families 4.85 billion $US in compensation without admitting any guilt (157). It is important to understand the size of these pharmaceutical giant companies with hundreds of thousands of employees, for which 5 billion dollars just is one fast move to the pocket book.

Many physicians and researches have defended this company saying that this is simply what happens in the RCTs. It is impossible to identify all adverse effects. We need to see this as times goes by, and then, if the drugs are not OK, withdraw them. It can't be done in any other way. The argument is valid. But only if the pharmaceutical companies follow the drugs in the intent of finding the adverse effects. In the case of Vioxx many people got the opposite impression: That the company tried to hide the deadly adverse effects for the public to keep the drug on the marked, and e-mails was even found where employees in the company had made hit lists of researchers on Vioxx' adverse effects who were to be discredited and destroyed (157). This impression was helped by email read in the court saying things like: "We may need to seek them out and destroy them where they live" (157). Most medical researchers do not like it when the pharmaceutical industry acts this way. We get somewhat nervous. Big Pharma is a little too big for this game to be funny.

When the drug hits the market we get one more opportunity to monitor the true, un-manipulated effect of the drugs, and the public health systems could easily do that. Again, this is not done. The physicians are formally required to rapport all suspect adverse effects, but during our obligatory medical training as a GPs, working in a large clinic with many other physicians we never heard of one physician filling in one single adverse-reaction-scheme. This was the only thing we could do as physicians we were are not paid to do. So as the other GPs we did do not do it. We did not even look for adverse effects. Or think about that the patients problems could be caused by the drugs. We simply treated whatever symptom, we found in the patient, until they had a drug for each organ system. Then there was not more we could do. Sometimes the patients went to the hospital, who cancelled all the medicine. Then we could start all over again.

Evaluation of Total Effect - Positive and Negative Effects All Together

The most important reasons for the pharmaceutical industry *not* using global self-rated questionnaire measuring the patient's quality of life, health and ability, is that this measure is *integrative*. It integrates the positive and the negative effects into a total measure of effect, where the positive effects the patient gets from a drug is balanced by the negative (237). In this simple way the total effect of a drug on a patient can be known. But this combined evaluation is NEVER done, as the pharmaceutical industry is not interested in all in combining the positive and the negative effects; this measure is only in the patients and his/her physician's interest. So the industry never measure that.

The basic strategy of evaluation is the other way round: It is very important to separate the good and the bad outcomes for only in this way can the industry claim its fine results. The adverse effects are hidden as well as possible, and what are left are all the positive helpful qualities of the new, commercial drugs. The game is understandable; make a double account where the loss is in one account and the gain is in another, and lose the first. Then everything looks nice and pink. Then the patient and the physician will believe that the drug helps. Because they want to believe that. Then there is hope, isn't there? Is it deception? Is if fraud? Yes it is. Do you think the pharmaceutical industry by accident made the RCT test separate positive and negative outcome and lose the negative? Well, if you do, think again.

Our problem is not in understanding the pharmaceutical industry; it wants to make money, that's the name of the game. Our problem lies in understanding all the national organs controlling the research and controlling medicine. These people, hired by the state to take care of the patients' interest, are systematically behaving as they were employed by Big Pharma. Maybe they are. Why would they behave like that if they weren't? We are sure these people are not as most of them having both an MD and a PhD are not stupid. The must know. Every single book keeper in this world knows this simple trick.

What is the consequence for the patients? Well, as the RCT secures that almost all pharmaceutical drugs on the market are strongly poisonous, this way of counting secures that the gate is open for commercial use. If you could not document they were different from placebo AND better, there would be no commercial point, would there?

What are the consequences of the drugs being tested this way? Basically that poison is sold as medicine and that millions of patients in the western world now suffer severe harm from poisoning, as we shall see in chapter 8. Even worse, the worse consequence of having all these drugs falsely documented as helpful is that it makes the patient and his/her doctor believe, that there is a biochemical cure when there really isn't. Being in this believe the patients stays with the biomedical physician who really only has like on chance in a hundred to help, as we shall see in Chapter 6. Half the Danes are chronic patients now. And the health budgets explode as the drug companies continue to develop new drugs, and the physicians continue to give more and still more drugs to the patients. The burden of poisoning is taking the whole population down. It is indisputable that this is the way it is going with public health. If you wonder why this is not strange. Half the population is poisoned by the pharmaceutical industry. Thousands of the most poisonous drugs chemistry has ever made are generously distributed to the people. The new market is the kids with ADHD. For Gods sake. Safe you kids from these drugs.

By the way a fun story. We know from contact with people in the Danish Television that one of the companies that make these drugs tried to hide the fact that it was the drug company who had paid the research documenting the positive effect in RCTs on kids with ADHD. A parent took the company to the high court of Sweden and won the case, so she was allowed to see the files on the documentation that was kept secret. The day after burned the building with all the papers about the documentation, by accident of course (236). The drugs stayed on the market, and now one in three of the boys in fundamentally school in Skåne, southern Sweden, are on this drug. The school is made for the girls, and if the boys don't like it, let's drug them into passivity. Then they will be good and obedient citizens when they grow up. And good customers. Good thinking, Big Pharma.

But in reality you should not blame the pharmaceutical industry for trying to make money; this is their job. It is really the politicians who are completely occupied with materialistic wealth, who is responsible for the misery. Instead of focusing on the happiness and quality of life of the population they think about their own political carreer. And if you got strong alliances with the industry, you will always have money, power, media-access and enough to win the elections. And no industry is stronger than Big Pharma. But who are voting by the way? Maybe you need to think about this next time there is an election.

WHERE DOES ALL THIS LEAD US?

First we have seen that the RCT test has given all drugs "pass de libre" to the market as the comparison with placebo is no comparison at all. The we have seen that the secret of the RTC really is to use poisonous drugs as they always will come out better that the inert piece of chalk the pharmaceutical companies have called placebo. Finally we have now seen how poisonous drugs are made look beneficial and harmless. This is really smart. The pharmaceutical industry has found a golden egg. Any poison will be made into medicine.

To get the drugs approved you must 1) Hire a chemist who can make a new sufficiently poisonous designer drug to you (he just needs to modify one of the existent drugs a little, it does not take a big brain!) and take the patent (now this is your drug!) 2) then you use the smart scientific set up of the standard RCT, with passive placebo and some local outcome measures of positive effects (preferably a biochemical disease marker with as far relation to the patients clinical reality as possible) and a standard list over adverse effects. 3) Then send it to the local *Scientific Ethical Committee* (what a name! soo Big Pharma) where all your biomedically trained friends are waiting for it, to get an easy, fast and uncritical approval of the project. 4) Then run the clinical experiment where you make sure that everybody is paid, the patients, the doctors, the nurses, the hospitals, the universities. Be sure to involve hundreds of physicians and thousands of patients, who will be the ambassadors of the product in the end of the study. 5) Publish the results in a medical RCT journal. Don't you worry; if you used the RCT-test your paper will get published. 6) Send this documentation to your national health authorities for another fast and dirty approval to sell it on the market, and 7) Hire a task force of marketing people to help you collect your one billion US$.

It's not that difficult. Anybody who have read this book and have a medium brain capacity can make his own medical company. Just remember to be generous with your money. And stay friends with Big Pharma. That's important. Only take half or even less for yourself. Success takes sharing.

CONCLUSION

We have seen in this chapter that if you are clever and keep your outcomes local, you will be able to make a list of positive and a list of negative effects, to be kept separated. If you explode your list of negative outcomes into a thousand concrete events, all the Number Needed to Harm's (NNHs) will look large, and the drug will look safe. If you add all these small NNHs up to the total likelihood of getting an adverse effect, the NNH_{total} will of course be much smaller, and the drug will appear more poisonous. Often the NNH_{total} is about 1, meaning that all patients will get adverse effects, in spite of the NNH-numbers given by the pharmaceutical companies being much larger. New drugs look safer and more efficient than old drugs, but in most cases they are not. They are just tested smarter.

If you measure the global outcomes, like self-assessed health, quality of life, and ability, negative and positive effects cannot be separated, but will be added to an integrated measure of the total impact of the drug on the patient. If you are a pharmaceutical company, you will never do that.

A drug needs to be poisonous to create an active placebo effect to pass the RCT test. So choosing a poisonous drug is essential for producing the documentation of a new drugs being documented helpful. Using the right outcome measures for the adverse effects is essential for documenting that the drug is not so harmful that it really matters, so the drug can get approved and sold.

The reader is now supposed to be so familiar with the RCT that he or she can make his/her own pharmaceutical company. The RCT is really a golden egg. You can only win. Dont worry about a thing. Being a member of Big Pharma is easy. Piece of cake.

Now you may start wondering how to spend your first billion of dollars. But don't you worry about that. You'll manage. In reality you won't have sufficient time in this life-time to spend that kind of money, but then you can take care of your kids and your friends also, which is very nice. Now you are the true king of the capitalistic world. And everything (except happiness, love and health) can be bought for money. Just enjoy your life.

Chapter 5

THE OBSERVATION TIME OF THE RANDOMISED CLINICAL TRIAL (RCT)

The fourth and last part of our critique of the pharmaceutical companies' standard RCT-procedure is about the test times used. This point looks innocent, but it is not.

In our discussion of the active placebo effect we learned that a medical intervention with an active placebo drug usually has two phases: An active placebo phase, and a toxic phase. First the patient feels the change in his or her whole system, and subconsciously uses the occasion to change his/her attitudes and believes from the more negative to the more positive. This is the active placebo effects.

Then, if the patient stays on the toxic drug, he or she must pay the prize of relying on taking a toxic substance. The poisonous effect will dominate and this phase is therefore called the toxic phase. The art of classical, western allopathic medicine that used extremely toxic drugs like strychnine for healing, was to give a strong blow to the patients consciousness of short duration, and withdraw the treatment before the patient was harmed. This makes good sense to us. Pre-moderne medicine men and shamans did the same using the hallucinogenic drugs that only have the active placebo effect, and almost no toxic effects (122).

But modern medicine use active placebo drugs in another way. Now the physician is no longer in charge of medicine; the pharmaceutical companies have taken over. The RTC procedure turns strong poisons into medicine, not to be used as hit-and-run active placebo drugs, but to be used constantly and daily for a prolonged period of time. The active placebo effect is still the active principle but it is turned down so that it is harder to observe and less obvious. The reason for pharmacological medicine evolving into this kind of medicine is not so strange; there are obvious commercial interests in this. Chemical medicine must be a pill you take three times a day or so, to be a good commercial product. You cannot make much money on a hit-and-run effect. You need to make it into a product the patients will have to take for an extended span of time, presumably for the rest of the life. This is a good product. This is good money.

To make physicians and their patients accepts pharmaceuticals to be taken daily, the pharmaceutical industry had to create more scientific and less woo doo-like explanations to the active mechanism of medicine than "active placebo". The researchers of the industry and their collaborators in academic medicine worldwide therefore started an intensive research in the biochemical mechanism of disease, and our knowledge of biochemistry, DNA and chromosomes exploded. A strong interest came in genetics because if one could prove a disease to be genetic, this would most certainly mean a biochemical basis for this disease and possibly also a chemical cure. Chemical and chromosomal theories exploded for schizophrenia, depression, cancer, heart conditions etc. Huge research projects like the human genome project were started. But nothing substantial was found; in reality the many billions of dollars were just wasted. Only a few weak disease markers were found, which in the end did not have the power to explain much.

Twin studies showed that mono-zygote twins who were adopted early in life still had a concordance of 0.25-0.5 for schizophrenia, meaning that if one twin had schizophrenia, the other twin would also have it in 25-50% of cases (101,102). The problem with this research was that its results could as well be taken as proof for the opposite position: That psychosocial factors in the womb and in infancy was the critical factors for developing schizophrenia, which was the position of Freud, Jung, Reich, Grof and the other psychoanalysts, as this was what they found through their clinical experience (175).

As these things could not be decided based on facts the whole thing turned into a war of opinions, which is where medicine still stands today. The whole human gene project, costing billions of dollars, did not lead to the discovery of "the gene for schizophrenia" or "the gene for breast cancer". But now we have looked carefully for it and this gives us reason to believe that the chemical hypothesis of the diseases is wrong in its basis (101,102).

But by making chemical medicine less obviously active placebo and more founded in a diversity of medical hypothesis, the pharmaceutical companies tricked the doctors to forget about the active placebo effect, and starting to believe in neuro-chemical hypotheses for mental disorders etc. The pharmaceutical companies admittedly also reduced the doses of poison so they became less toxic that the hit-and-run allopathic doctors over-whelming doses of medicine. There are many stories about the allopathic doctors sometimes by accident killing the patient, which around 1900 invited a justified, hard critique of the allopathic doctors from their holistic and homeopathic colleagues. Its more gentle way spoke to the allopathic doctors who gradually became the biomedical doctors.

The problem is now: What if medicine still is basically about active placebo? What if all this fancy stories about correction the level of neurotransmitters in the brain etc is basically just stories with no scientific justification, i.e. not based on any scientific evidence? We have examined the rationale of the two most popular chemical hypothesis in psychiatry and found these not to be based on evidence (101). And the Cochrane metaanalysis of anti-depressant drugs vs. active placebo showed the effects of these drugs to be caused by active placebo[132]. So there we are. The hypothesis were just hypothesis that should help market the drugs. The physicians and the patients were all tricked by the stories and the RCT-based documentation. But is was and it stays active placebo medicine. Poisons, nothing else. The allopathic doctors who eagerly wanted to be the scientific doctors, are still the allopathic doctors.

Therefore the drug effects must be measured accordingly. The effect of the drug in the active placebo phase must be measured, and the effect of the drug in the toxic phase must be measured. Short-term effects and adverse effects must be measured, and long term effects and adverse effects must be measured.

At this point we are sure the reader has guessed our critique: The adverse effects are almost never measured in the long term. The pharmaceutical companies measure only adverse effects in the short term. In this period there is a strong active placebo effect and therefore few side effects. And when the active placebo effect goes down and the toxic effects of the drugs becomes manifest, the measuring stops.

So the way the pharmaceutical industry documents the effects of the drugs fits perfectly to the rest of the pattern: The effects are measured in such a time scale that the toxic effects are being hidden.

The adverse effects are typically measured for three month only, or even less, for the psychiatric drugs (81,133). But the patients are supposed to take them for life. This is not good. From our knowledge from standard toxicology we must suspect many toxic effects to accumulate though time. From other sources of data than the pharmaceutical companies we know that there are lots of harm to psychiatric patients taking these drugs for extended periods of time, like drug induced depressions (134), high frequency of suicide (210,211), and more spontaneous unexplained deaths than in people not taking these drugs (209). It is very bad that the pharmaceutical industry gets away with not documenting the adverse effects of the drugs though time. In this way strongly poisonous drugs are made look beneficial to the patients and their doctors, which these drugs judged from lots of evidence produced by independent researchers most obviously are not (81,133,135).

In general there is very few data on the long-term effects of the positive effects also; we have found data for the antipsychotic drugs indicating that the positive effect found on patients “global state” (“global impression”) goes down from NNT=4 in short term to NNT=7 in the intermediate term, for thereafter presumably to disappear completely (no data!) (81,158).

In general it is unacceptable to let the patients take an active placebo drug, which essentially is only a poison without any specific positive, pharmacological action, for more than a very short period of time.

But the good business is to make everybody believe that the drugs has a good and permanent effect, and should be taken for years and years. To sell the drugs that would only be used for a week would not make much of a profit, would it?

The long-term adverse effects of antipsychotic drugs are seen at the many institutions for mentally ill. Often there is a complete loss of ability to study and work, a loss of social network and social abilities, loss of libido and sexual desire, loss of alertness and ability to concentrate, a dramatically increased number of physical health problems (81), and as mentioned above a dramatically increased tendency of suicide with 15% of the patients committing suicide in Denmark (210,211), and a 50% over-mortality when the antipsychotic drugs are combined with other drugs, what they often are (209).

No wonder that these patients after 10 years of medication often look more like vegetables than men. The drugs are in reality killing them, depraving them of their beautiful you lives, which according to statistics from treatment of holistic medicine often could be improved (58,80,109-111,113).

CONCLUSION

The pharmaceutical industry insists that the randomised clinical trial be used to test the chemical medicine, in spite of this test having four fundamental errors that complement each other in such a way that they together give the RCT test a fatal error: It makes poison into medicine.

The chemical medicine is not tested against placebo, as the "placebo pill" has no placebo effect at all. All biologically active drugs are poisonous and the more poisonous a drug is, the more will it be favored by the RTC test. The way the effects are measured are ingeniously efficient in hiding the poisonous effect of the poisonous drugs, and the time frame used for the testing is as if the designer of the test exactly knew what timeframe would give the best results.

The outcome measures are most often not clinically relevant and the only really meaningful measure, the global quality of life, which could show if there really was a benefit for the patient in taking the drug, is never used. Self-assessed health, the strongest known predictor of future survival and healthy is not measured either. The RCTs are not using clinically relevant outcome measures as clinical benefits for the patients are not the goal of the production of the chemical medicine. It is only about money.

The RCT test pretends to be blind. It is not. It pretends to be scientific. It most definitely is not. It pretends to document the scientific value of a pharmaceutical drug, but it only documents the value of the drugs as short term active placebo drugs. If the doctors knew of this function they might be used in this way, but the physicians has come to believe in the hypothesis so often repeated by the industry and its allies that they almost have become scientific truths.

The hypotheses about the drugs are as smart justifications for the drugs but they are not at all substantiated. These hypotheses seem to be created by helpful academics serving the pharmaceutical industry.

The pharmaceutical industry has succeeded in making so many good doctors and their patients believe in drugs. They believe that the drugs are based on hard-core scientific theory. They believe the chemical medicine to be evidence-based because of the RCTs. They have been deceived. Badly.

The RCT-test as it is today, measuring against nothing, hiding its use of active placebo, measuring in clinically meaningless dimensions and neglecting all long-term effects of the drugs, is in no way useable for scientific testing of pharmaceuticals. It is not a scientific test. It is a scamp. It is a fraud. It is a trick. It does not at all do what it is supposed to do. It turns the most poisonous highly biologically active substances known to the world today into seemingly useful chemical medicine. If you take the drugs tested with the RCT test you are most likely to get poisoned, not to get cured. In spite the labels of the pharmaceutical drugs telling you the opposite.

The public health authority, who is obliged to control the medicine, has been sleeping in the hour. The physicians and their patients have been deceived.

It is our belief that the pharmaceutical industry intentionally has twisted the RCT-test to maximize its own profit. With the flawed RCT-test it can take any strong poison and document it to be useful medicine, with a high efficacy and only modest harm. The RCT makes strong poisons that never should enter a human body into highly profitable medical products, which the most vulnerable and trusting, ill people then are getting from the person they need to trust the most: His or her own doctor.

In a historic victory over the classical holistic medicine, the pharmaceutical industry has managed to substitute the old psychosocial medicine, the holistic medicine of Hippocrates, which has been the acknowledged European medicine for over 2000 years, with thousands of poisonous chemical substances, that we have no reason at all to believe should have specific pharmacological beneficial effects. They only test positive in the RCT test because they are poisonous. And that's it.

This fraud, this criminal act of stealing medicine from society to make transform it into a cold business, that only can harm the patients, is truly a disaster for mankind. We have collectively lost the precious gem of medicine on the floor.

Sick people can no longer get help from their doctor who has lost faith in loving care and psychosocial interventions and now only believes in chemistry. The patients can no longer get a healing cure from their physician. As a result the patients stay ill, and become chronically ill patients. According to the statistics they stay ill forever, and in Denmark where socialized medicine is totally dominated by biomedicine every second citizen is a chronic patient now (2). Medicine does not cure any longer. It has been kidnapped. Hijacked. It has been raped, abducted, humiliated, and destroyed.

Medicine does not heal its patients any more. We have known this for a long time in Denmark. Now we also know why. It was for the money.

Chapter 6

EFFICACY OF BIOMEDICINE IN GENERAL PRACTICE: WHY ONLY ONE PATIENT IN A HUNDRED GETS HELP

In the rich and happy country of Denmark – for many years the richest in the world - well, not as happy as people outside Denmark normally think, more *satisfied* with everything because of our social stability, we are so lucky that we have *socialized medicine* (159).

We have socialized medicine in the sense that we have *socialized biomedicine*, meaning that as a lucky citizen of Denmark you can get free biomedical treatment. You can see your biomedical doctor (but not your holistic doctor) as often as you like, and you don't have to pay. Drugs are not totally free, but almost because they are subsidized by the government, and if your medicine is expensive (more than 350 USD a year) or if you are a chronic patient the state will subsidize most of it or even often it all. If you cannot afford the drugs, and are on social benefits, the country will pay it all for you. In reality this means free biomedicine – all the pharmaceutical drugs you want – for everybody, for as long as you live.

Half of the Danish population is chronically ill (2), and for most of these patients it means taking a drug constantly, every day, for many years. At least one in four suffers from chronic pain[2]. But many more patients than the chronically ill feel bad and they also go to their physician. Most of these people will also get drugs in spite of not being ill. So most of the Danes, sick or not, uses drugs: Pain killers, sleeping pills, anti-depressive drugs, anti-anxiety drugs, anti-psychotic drugs etc.

Socialized medicine seems a wonderful idea. The sick, the week, and the poor have free admission to medical care, free hospitals, free immunizations, free medical examinations, blood tests, X-rays, CT-scans etc. 50 billion DKR pr. Years or 3.500 USD per chronic patient, is used for this every year – paid by tax money (the rich people pay about 70% of the last money they make in Denmark as tax).

This socially oriented Danish society makes the rich pay, but we like it anyway. We Danes love Denmark, very much the same way Americans love America and Germans love Germany. But many more people love socialized medicine. President Obama wants it for the USA. Health is important after all, isn't it?

In Denmark we have *holistic* and *alternative* medicine also, often called CAM, integrative or psychosocial medicine. As has the USA. But this you have to pay for yourself in Denmark. Why non-drug medicine in general is *not* covered by the national medical insurance is not so clear. The official story is that Denmark only covers *evidence based medicine*, based on RCTs. In reality this is not true because many nationally supported drugs have never been thoroughly documented in RCTs, so it is all about politics.

The more authoritarian a system you have in your country, the fewer people hold the power, and the easier it is for the industry to lobby the system. So basically Big Pharma has won the battle about Denmark: Socialized medicine has come to mean ONLY biomedicine.

In USA this is different. The American citizen has to pay for medicine him or herself, and already about 1990 this meant that the money spent on CAM in America is much more than the money spent on biomedicine. Also, biomedicine happens to cost about 10 times as much in US than in Denmark. In Denmark a bed for 24 hours at a biomedical hospital usually cost about 5000 DKR (800 USD); in USA the same bed often costs 6000 USD. Why this is so is not clear; the official explanation is that insurance is so high because of a million medical lawsuits. In Denmark you cannot get money by suing a doctor. But to make a long story short, America loves CAM, and much more money goes to CAM than to biomedicine (61,162).

In Denmark more and more people want holistic and alternative medical treatment, with 10% of the population using it in 1990, 20% using CAM in 2000 (160) and this development seems to continue reaching a fraction of about 40% using CAM in 2010. In 10 years or so Denmark will shift to CAM, if the pharmaceutical industry does not manage to stop the development. But biomedicine reacts to this threat. We have seen biomedical doctors being more and more aggressive towards the holistic health care providers and researchers during the last 10 years (70).

The important thing to notice here is that this development towards holistic non-drug medicine is happening in spite of biomedicine being free for everybody and CAM costing 100 USD per hour. So what is happening here? Everybody seems to realize that free biomedicine has turned 50% or so of the population into chronic patients and very often even dependent drug abusers. Biomedicine does not work: It does not cure the people.

In Denmark we have had this grand scale experiment with free biomedicine on behalf of the world. So now we know how things will develop if you choose biomedicine as your basic medical system in your society. Every second person will become a chronically ill patient. Half of these people cannot even work: the other part has a severely compromised quality of life (42,43).

Why then are the Danes the happiest people in the world? Because everybody feels supported and safe. If you are ill and unable to work, the state will give you medical treatments and also social benefits for life. Everybody has a nice home. And even the poorest has a car. If you are chronically ill you will also have a free parking lot close to your door. And a nice TV set. And you will be able to buy fine organic food from great Danish farms. What more can you expect from life?

When you have what you go for, you are happy. Well, not really happy in the deep existential sense which nobody seems to care about, but pretty satisfied with your life as a whole. 15 years ago our research team has documented that the Danish people are not really happy, in the deep existential sense of being realized and enlightened beings. But we are happy in the sense of being very satisfied. Like people are just after a huge meal. Are you happy? Oh yes, thank you, I couldn't take another bite! That kind of happiness.

So while Denmark is shifting away from biomedicine, being the world's first country to offer that to the people, the rest of the world is going Denmark's way. But is this a good idea? Shouldn't we learn a little from the experiences of Denmark?

One of the severe problems connected to biomedicine is that everybody treated with pharmaceutical drugs is learning a specific understanding of health and disease, the biomedical understanding. It is a mechanical understanding putting a lot of weight on genes and DNA, and brain chemistry and a lot of hypothesis with little foundation in facts (101). And the education to this mechanical world view starts the first moment you are treated by a doctor and gets a drug, normally penicillin for acute otitis or a similar infection, as a child.

In holistic medical science this side effect of treatment, that you change your beliefs, is called "implanted philosophy". The place where this is mostly happening is within psychiatry where the patents are talked into believing in the chemical ideas of life by their psychiatrist. Coercive persuasion is often used to make the patients accept these ideas (136).

Talking of treating children it is worth noticing that penicillin hardly makes a different in children; a Cochrane metaanalysis of the treatment of acute otitis documented that this treatment doesn't prevent loss of hearing; for one in fifteen (NNT=15) the pain is little less after the treatment, but for every child the administration of penicillin is in itself a burden. Every father and mother knows that. In spite of no scientific rationale 98% of all children in USA get penicillin for acute otitis (163).

The Cochrane researchers explain that many of the children get adverse effects of the drug. How many children that develop allergy to penicillin because of this early and unnecessary treatment is not known, but we know that it is often very difficult to treat adult patients who are allergic to penicillin. Most likely the treatment with penicillin for diseases that are easily cured by the patient own immune system makes much more harm than good. In principle most physicians agree on that. But when the mother sits there begging for penicillin to her sick child it takes a hard heart not to make the prescription. Besides, it is good money. A doctor also needs to earn a living, right?

In general biomedical treatments are not based on science as we have seen; they are - in spite of what most physicians believe - not *evidence-based* at all. This is what the pharmaceutical industry wants your doctor and you as a costumer to believe, for you to buy the drugs.

The Danes has had a strong belief in the "magic bullet". A strong belief in science and progress. A belief in rationality, and in social welfare. 10 years ago the quality of life revolution rolled over the country. This was a philosophical movement that thought every Dane that happiness and health came from self-insight and wise use of personal resources, and not from money, education, social status etc.

Basically the message was identical with the teaching of the old Hippocratic doctors: Meaning of life is what matters. Since then, biomedicine has had a hard time in the public opinion. But the pharmaceutical industry has understood to use the doctors and to lobby towards the government to keep the biomedical health system intact. So the castle of socialized biomedicine is still standing. It will fall. We think in a few years from now. Because the Danes read newspapers and books, like the one you are reading now.

How many patients are helped by the holistic general practitioner?

To be honest, we don't know. We have done research in CAM, with cranio-sacral therapy and other types of CAM for whiplash, together with the University Hospital at Odense, and found that this kind of therapy did not work at al. At that point in time we were strong believers in CAM, but the negative results from our own research changed that. We have decently published the negative results from our CAM-study (244).

Other researcher in CAM has found acupuncture, homeopathy, individualized herbal treatments (170) etc not to be very effective. We know that every year in Denmark we get a thousand or so know new CAM-therapists practicing these inefficient types of medicine; we also know that the general health of the Danish population is deteriorating, meaning that all these thousands of CAM therapists, living from treating about two millions of chronic patients dissatisfied with the efficacy of the biomedical drugs that does not cure them, are not curing them either[2]. CAM is today in Denmark delivered as a supplement to the established biomedical treatment. So in fact most of the chronically ill patients get the drug-CAM combination that does not help them. That does not help.

But the classical, holistic medicine is very different from this kind of CAM. It is build on a completely different philosophy of life and it does not mix with the mechanical worldview of patients, meaning that if you want to be treated successfully by holistic medicine you need to be aware of your worldview and choose side. Materialism or spiritualism. Matter or consciousness. Money or love. Basically.

The classical holistic doctor did not use any drugs. The Hippocratic medicine has from its earliest days been a strict non-drug medicine (3,122-128). The Hippocratic doctor's tools have been talk and touch therapy. His single aim has been to help the patient explore him-self to understand life, body, disease, self, sexuality, character etc better. In the self-exploration was the key to understanding the disease and though this understanding came the healing about.

As everybody *in principle* can be helped to higher self- insight holistic medicine is really a tool that *in principle* can help everybody. It is often called clinical medicine (100); in the tradition of clinical medicine the cure is the thorough assisted examination of the problems, eventually leading to the answers. In the tradition of clinical medicine all patients has the same basic problem: Lack of self-insight. Therefore every patient is treated very much the same way, making thorough diagnoses and medical examinations much less relevant than the exploration of the experienced problems here and now, in body and mind, together with the patient (164).

Independent of the patients suffering from a physical or mental disorder, an existential, psychological sexual, or social problem, supported self-exploration is the key to personal development, improvement of quality of life and health, and in the end to better use of all the persons talents, making him a much more happy and contributing citizens.

So how effective is holistic medicine? Well, since 1997 we (SV) has run the Research Clinic for Holistic Medicine and Sexology, as described in a number of books (34,35,37-39), papers (15,19,62,112-117) and case stories (see15). we have with our own eyes seen the majority of patients (NNT=2), independently of the problem they presented, be cured just from engaging in personal development under our leadership, making them assume responsibility and gain self-insight in our own clinic. We have even miraculously seen patients even with schizophrenia and cancer occasionally be well again as reported in our papers (192,200). And we have seen no adverse effects (15).

But we have to admit that the patients normally came to us after reading our popular books on quality of life and consciousness-based holistic medicine. They knew who we were and what we believed in. They know what we were up to. So our patients have been highly selected.

In general, all patients from research in holistic medicine, the cancer patients of Dr. David Spiegel or the heart patients of Dr. Dean Ornish, has volunteered to the treatment, after informed consent which is thorough information giving the patients a good understanding the ideas and principles of the treatment. The patients have all been exceptional in some way. They were looking for an alternative cure themselves. They had assumed responsibility. They were not normal patients. They believed. They reached out. They got cured because of this.

It's even hard to tell what would have happened if we had not offered all these patients a holistic treatment. I guess many of them would have found another person to help them. Maybe even not a doctor. They had the will to live, and the will to come back to life. In my opinion this was what helped them. Nor our brilliant expertise.

So maybe the universe is perfect as it is. The people who need to get cured find an excuse to heal. And the people who need to stay ill will find an excuse to stay ill. The first group will go to the holistic doctors that help them explore life and develop as persons. The latter group will find a biomedical physician, take drugs for years, and stay ill.

In a way this philosophical position is a little too pessimistic for our taste. We believe that a good physician can and will make a difference for the patient. The doctor is the tool[129]. The doctor is like the loving father, or the good friend, who can be there for you and give you the support and loving care you need to heal. The doctor is important. Very much so.

Symptomatic treatment with drugs and the biomedical physician believing in it cannot offer the suffering people of the world loving support and self exploration. It might seem so at a first glance, but this is just façade. The energy is channeled in another direction, away from confronting and solving the problems.

Biomedicine offers fear, closed eyes, hope of betterment that only the physician and his drugs can fulfill (but almost never will), low responsibility for own life and existence… Basically biomedicine offers a more mechanical and materialistic world view, where man is seen more as a victim than as a worrier. More like a chemical machine than as a divine, living being.

To conclude this section all available statistics, from our own clinic and from other fine clinics mostly in Sweden, England, Germany and the USA (109), has shown that one patient in two or more are cured with holistic medicine. Not helped. Cured. Improved to a state where they no longer feel ill (62,112-117). But all these patients have been highly selected – by themselves – before the treatment. They have had a strong will to get well, to improve and to win the battle of life. We know from Danish research by Ulrik Dige that this is what it takes to win even over you cancer (get spontaneous remission) (245). If you believe strong enough you can just go to Sai Baba in India to get cured (120). We (SV) were there. It seemed to work.

So holistic medicine is extremely efficient if you can accept the idea that the disease is caused by lack of self-insight and at poor quality of life in the first place. If you believe that disease is caused by genes, DNA, and chemistry, you are not likely to not benefit much from holistic treatment. Because you would not go to a holistic doctor in the first place. In Chapter 7 we will give you the detailed statistics of holistic medicine. We will not repeat that we believe that it is the patients that cure themselves. Not us that cures them. But we do believe that.

HOW MANY PATIENTS ARE HELPED BY THE BIOMEDICAL GENERAL PRACTITIONER?

For the biomedical GP the situation is very different than for the holistic doctor, who just can start treating the patient right away, from the first moment of the first meeting. First you cannot as a biomedical physician treat any patient without being certain of the diagnosis. To establish this often takes time, weeks or even months, and often lots of blood- and tissue samples, bacterial cultures, microscopy and hospital lab analyses. Often in more complicated cases it takes several months to establish the correct diagnosis. The patient has to wait for the treatment to begin.

If the patient only suffers from existential or minor mental and psychological problems like personality disturbances, character problems, disturbances of social function, sexual problems etc. there will in most cases be no biomedical treatment (109-111).

Chronic pains without a biological cause cannot be treated successfully in the biomedical clinic and one Dane in five suffers from chronic pain (2). Of course there are painkillers, on paper very efficient, but in reality there are no scientific reasons to believe that painkillers like the very popular NSAIDs should help the chronic pain patients at all (67). If people believe they help they will take them. Patients do rarely make the experiment to measure their quality of life and health with and without the drugs. Without rigid psychometric tools such experiments are prone to so much bias that they become of no value, and even the smart patients realize that. We need science to tell us if this is good for us. We rely on science. We have to.

People who come to their GP because they feel that they lack energy, just feel bad, dizzy, slightly disoriented, without really being ill, cannot be helped by drugs. If the quality of life is low and there is nothing wrong with body and mind, the biomedical doctor can do little about it. There simply are no drugs that can improve the general quality of life!

On the other hand, if you are really ill, physically or mentally, with schizophrenia, a bad heart or most types of cancers, there is no successful cure either (82-85,132,133). Chemical medicine can hardly make any difference here; well, according to the statistics presented in detail below, the pharmaceutical drugs are likely to harm you much more than they benefit, destroy your quality of life, and shorten your life.

If the patient suffers from a disease that can be treated rationally with chemical medicine, the treatment can only be successful with the correct diagnosis, but only about two in three gets this, and the rest will get drugs for an irrelevant disease (246-294). Patients who get the wrong diagnosis are not likely to benefit from the treatment as they get the wrong drug (or the wrong dose) but they will still get the adverse effects of the drugs taken.

Even with the correct diagnosis many patients get the wrong treatment (246-294); a too high or too low dose or simply a wrong drug. In Denmark we have been very surprised to learn how many patients that gets the wrong drug by accident, either because the prescription is incorrect, or because the nurses or pharmacists giving the drugs are making mistakes (246-294). If the disease is treatable, correctly diagnosed, and the patient is given the correct medicine in the correct dose (at the correct time), we know that about one patient in three do not take the medicine as they should (110). This is called low compliance. The patients forget, or they don't like the adverse effects so they reduce dose, or they even switch the drugs with their friends to take drugs they feel more appropriate. Many patients, who become dependent of the drugs, ask their doctor for as strong drugs as they can get, then sell the drugs on the black market and buy new stronger ones instead. Patients prostitute themselves to get the dope. Many patients drink alcohol with the drugs to increase or modify their effect. This is clearly a mess. In the end only one in ten or so of the patients gets the correct drugs for the correct, treatable disease, and use the drugs as prescribed (110,164).

And now, it is time to recall that the Number Needed to Treat (the NNT-number) is about 20 for most types of pharmaceutical drugs (79). Let's forget here that many of the modern drugs do not even use clinically relevant outcomes, making this number even less. And let's forget the problems with the RCTs mentioned about making even the drugs' ability to help this limited number very doubtful. Let play along with the rules of biomedicine, and accept the NNT=20. Then we know that only one in 200, or 0.5% of these patients are helped (110). The 199 patients that are not helped become chronic patients. Like most of the patients that becomes helped but not cured.

It is not difficult to see why most patients end up as chronic patients. If you are not sick, but think you are, you will feel chronically ill, in spite of your doctor insisting on you being completely well. If you are incurably ill you will, stay ill. And if you are in the lucky third or so that in principles could be helped, you most likely will not be. This is the reason that on in two of the Danes these days are chronic patients.

Biomedicine can simply not keep a population healthy. But everybody will take drugs, and continue to do this for the rest of their lives. Which is why biomedicine is the most profitable business there is.

Let's see this in hard numbers: Of 100 patients going to the GP, 33 is not physically or mentally ill but has a psychological, existential or sexual problem, that cannot be solved though biomedicine and drugs. These are not helped. As these problems from a holistic-medical perspective are caused by lack of self-insight and bad use of personal resources, they could be solved with holistic medicine.

Of the remaining 67, 33 have a disease, but something that cannot be cured by today's biomedicine; these patients will remain chronically ill to the day, unless a miracle like spontaneous remission of cancer happens. As biomedicine is rather authoritarian many of these patients are likely to get the belief from their biomedical physician that they cannot be well again, and so they will not seek an alternative solution. A lot of these patients will at some point in time enter a CAM treatment; in Denmark we have about one reflexologist per 1000 citizens, and 3 other CAM-therapists per 1000 citizens, and half the patients uses their services as a complementary medicine to biomedicine, but the cocktail of biomedicine and CAM does not help them to be well again. The physicians offering holistic medicine, that really could help many of these patients, are not financially supported by the government so they are very few. The few there are struggling with attacks from the biomedical doctors as it happens all over the planet these years; they are systematically discredited in by their biomedical colleagues in the media, scaring many patients from using them. As a result these 33 stays ill.

- Of the remaining 34 that could be helped with biomedicine, 11 gets the wrong diagnosis, and hence the wrong drug.
- Of the remaining 23 at least 3 will get the wrong medicine or the correct medicine but in a wrong dose.
- Of the remaining 20, only 10 will take the medicine as prescribed (about half the patients in Denmark have low compliance).
- Of these remaining 10 patients, who in principle could be helped by the pharmaceutical drugs, at least according to the documentation based on the RCTs, one in twenty, in this example one patient max, will be helped (NNT=20). But rarely cured.

If we look at the side effects of the treatment, this is also a sad story. The biomedical physician gets paid to make a prescription. To do this is fast and easy. And almost always expected by the patient who have been to the doctor before, and who also got a prescription last time. So in practice almost every patient will get some chemical medicine. You can always try a mild anti-depressant (the patient seems a little depressed), a mild sedative (isn't there some anxiety there?), a sleeping pill (worries often keep people awake), and some innocent painkillers (problems almost always somatisize into some kind of pain, low back pain, stomach pain etc), and maybe some hormones for the females (if the periods are not regular, menopause is coming soon etc). These treatments are not scientifically justified , but the doctor's clinic is also a business, you shouldn't forget that, and if the physician wants to make his 150.000 USD a year or so, he really needs to get things rolling.

So let's return to the 100 patients. Of the 33 patients who are not ill, 3 will not be offered a prescription, 4 will refuse the prescription, and 26 will accept to get a prescription. Of the 33 who are incurably ill all will get a prescription. Of the 34 who are, in principle, curable, everybody will get a prescription. So of the 100 patients, 93 or so will get a prescription. About a quarter, or 23, of these patients will not take the drugs, because they don't believe them to help, or don't experience them to help if they start to take them. Another quarter will take them but not as prescribed, i.e. they will take tree pills in the morning instead of one three times a day, making the plasma level escalate to an extend where the drug to not work anymore. But one in three (NNH=3), or 8 of these patients will still get the adverse effects. Half, or 47 of the patients, will take the drugs as prescribed, and one in three (NNH=3), or 18 patients, will get significant adverse effects from the poisonous effects of the drugs.

So 70 patients will take the drugs, and of these 24 patients will and 46 patients will not get adverse effects, according to the documentation based on the RCTs.

But we know by now that the documentation of the adverse effects is made by the pharmaceutical companies, who often cheat to make their drugs look more efficient and less harmful. We know that minor side effects like dizziness, loss of concentration and libido, loss of memory and mental sharpness, loss of social ability and quality of life, is NOT documented. But what is more important, we know that all the adverse effects of the drugs only are documented short term, and that they might be much more dangerous in the long run, meaning that if patients take these drugs for years they might be seriously harmed, without anyone connecting this to the use of pharmaceutical drugs. But wake up. You take poisons – biologically active chemicals that everybody KNOWS are toxic – for years, so what do you expect? That organic milk, green salad, and bicycling can compensate for that???

So we find it fair to conclude that, based on the existing documentation from the pharmaceutical companies based on the RCT, that while one is helped by biomedicine, nobody is likely to be cured, and a quarter of all the patients attending the biomedical GPs office will get poisoned and harmed by the chemical medicine.

As the results from the industrial RCTs are strongly biased, reality is worse. As we doubt the RCT-based drug trials to be a scientific test, they way the RCTs are used today, but more a smart commercial for drugs, as Gøtzsche found in his doctoral thesis accepted by University of Copenhagen[67], we doubt that the one patient that should be helped, is really helped. We also doubt that the 46 patients taking the drugs without documented harm are not harmed. They are taking poison, why shouldn't this be harmful? Maybe you cannot see a specific damage to body or mind, but poisons will burden your organism and take your energy as your body has to deal with it. It might not cause permanent damage, as our bodies are extremely capable of healing itself, but is still causes imbalances and disturbances, that diminish your performance and your quality of life. You get a little more grey, low, tired and wearied out. See?

If a Danish patient is a chronically ill patient, this is because the drugs have not helped. The likelihood of a drug helping the patient now goes down from 5% (NNT=20) to maybe one percent (NNT=100). Nobody really knows that as this kind of sad and depressive research in the lack of therapeutic efficacy is almost never founded, and definitively not carried out by the pharmaceutical industry itself. But most chronic patients seem to stay chronic patients for life, in spite of continued biomedical treatment and this does not indicate a significant success rate for helping these patients.

CONCLUSION – HOW ARE THINGS IF WE ACCEPT THE VALIDITY OF THE RCTS FOR A MOMENT?

So let's conclude this section. In Denmark we have socialized medicine. Unfortunately the pharmaceutical industry has managed to repress holistic medicine to such an extent that holistic medicine is no longer supported financially by the government. Only if you want to practice biomedicine, you can get paid for treating you patients.

The system works in such a way that the physicians are paid per visit and per prescription, meaning that all visits should be short and all patients should have a prescription, for the doctor to be happy. This is a crazy system. You are allowed to have longer talks with a few patents each week. But you are not paid accordingly. If you want to make money, push drugs, drugs, and more drugs.

When we analyze the situation in detail, which we have done (110), we have found that only 10% or so of the patients use the drugs as indented, for the clinical conditions they are supposed to help for, and of these patients only one in 20 (NNT=20 in average for the pharmaceutical drugs (79)) or 0.5% is helped. These drugs rarely cure the patients; more often they just block symptoms.

At the same time, drugs are given to almost every patient, but only taken by about two third of the patients, or 70 patients in our example. Of these one in three, or 24 (NNH=3) will get adverse effects.

So even if we accept the industrial documentation based on the RCTs we find this: In total of a 100 patients, a maximum of 1 patient is helped by the drugs, while 24 get harmed. The doctor gets rich, the pharmaceutical companies overwhelmingly wealthy, and the people gets poisoned. Welcome to the brave, new world of biomedicine.

For the 95%, getting the correct diagnosis and treatment but who is not helped by the drugs, the NNT is of course much higher. We estimate NNT=100 for this group, but is could realistically very well be NNT=1000. All this is evaluated on the condition that the documentation from the RCT is actually valid.

BUT NOW, WHEN WE KNOW THE RCT IS NOT VALID, HOW ARE THINGS THEN?

Not much different. More patients' gets adverse effects, even less patients get helped. But the rationale for the whole circus has gone. This makes the beautiful young girls representing the medical companies and visiting the physicians' clinic every week to "inform about the new drugs" (often former chearleaders of course) look even more doubtful, and the biomedical physician believing in the drugs in the end look just like a fool.

It is no wonder that biomedical doctors burn out, as they often do. Suicide rate among biomedical physicians is sky high all over the world, which is quite understandable, as these people often see the same patients again and again and again, trying to give them a new drug and a new drug and a new drug, this going on for years and years. It is understandable that they feel that they create no value to the patients, and they often don't. If they are warm and caring human beings, which most doctors are in the beginning of their medical carrier, they will create value for their patients in the beginning, but as seeing a patent in 12.5 minute becomes routine, and the time for chat and small talk disappears, the doctors do not manage to come to know their patients on a personal level. Medical work becomes routine, the work gets speeded up, all justified by the scientific explanations attached to the drugs. More and more drugs are provided, less and less love and care, and in the end the physician feels this as a completely meaningless endeavor. And some kill themselves. This is understandable. Quite understandable.

Biomedicine has a fundamental problem it is worldview that is so much larger than just problems with the testing of the drugs. Biomedicine believes that life is chemistry. We don't. Of course we consist of atoms and molecules, but life is first of all about coherent fields of awareness and information, collected though billions of years that life has existed on this planet. And maybe there is information in the whole universe that is shared by all living beings, also. We don't know. But sometimes it feels like it.

Biomedicine comes from a mechanical worldview, chemistry. But it also comes from western industry. When medicine can be turned into a pill, and sold on small glasses and buckets and containers with great looking labels ensuring its efficacy and relative harmlessness, it becomes an outstanding business opportunity. All the ill and troubled people of the world want a fast and simple solution. They are caught in the commercial world, busy making a living, working at schools and at factories and shops, trying hard to survive, and living in more or less dysfunctional families. They are easily misinformed. They are so easily fooled by the smart guys in the pharmaceutical industry that even manage to fool their doctors, who are supposed to be smart. Well, who often is smarter than them, and in whom they trust. The doctor trusts the pharmaceutical industry. And the pharmaceutical industry screws them all.

The alternative to the mechanical world view is the spiritual world view. This is about love, about the magic of life. It's about consciousness, understanding, self-exploration, personal responsibility, ethics and so forth.

If the doctor comes from this he will understand the complexity of the patient's reality. Life is a spiritual journey, and everything is happening for the sake of learning and personal development. Diseases serve a purpose. They are here to teach us something. And something of great importance, something about the meaning of life. Diseases are invitations to look inside one self, and get an understanding of who we are and how we operate. Diseases are invitations to self-exploration, personal growth, and self-realization. This is the holistic physician's perspective, shared by so many doctors though the ages (3,6,12,16,19,37-39,46-58).

It is not so strange that it is difficult to make a correct biomedical diagnosis, for the diagnostic system does not really fit to the human being. The diagnostic system of biomedicine is itself developed to serve the purpose of helping the biomedical physician to give the correct drugs. While the patient almost always presents a multifaceted and complex problem (166-168), often with elements of existential problems, disturbed sexuality, somatisized pains, hypochondria, and many more problems coming from incomplete psychosexual development and unsatisfactory development of the personality and integrity (78), this picture is just very hard to call "anxiety", "depression" or "pain". These simple terms simply does not describe what is going in. If the physician is a person in personal development, the complexity of life and its deeper meaning will be appreciated in general, and the patient's problems make a lot of sense. Which basically is why the holistic physician can help his patients, and help most patients with most problems (109,111-119,121-129,165,169).

Another way to put it is that the holistic physician tries his best to help the patient to feel as a part of a larger wholeness, a welcomed member of the world. The goal is to induce a *sense of coherence* (SOC) in the patient. If the holistic physician succeeds the patient will heal not only mind, body, feelings, thoughts etc but his or her whole existence – a process called salutogenesis by the researcher Aron Antonovsky (155,156). Antonovsky's theory of existential healing is the first theory of its kind that has gained international recognition. Antonovsky managed to explain how the whole person could heal, not only his mind or body. When this happens everything else is improved: physical and mental health, quality of life, general ability in sexuality, work and social relations. To help the patient understand life and develop a new sense of coherence and meaning of life is the golden purpose of holistic medicine, as it has been for millennia since Hippocrates and his students 2400 years ago (3).

With its super aggressive marketing of biomedical drugs, often using illegal marketing [ref], and its widespread cooperation with the academic institutions about biomedical research, Big Pharma has succeeded in making the world forget the spirit of medicine, the essence of healing, and even the heart of man and the meaning of life itself.

The pharmaceutical industry has a tremendous impact on the world of today on a philosophical level, taking everything down to chemistry, taking the focus away from man and his reality, destroying the sense of coherence of the doctor as well as of his patients. The RCT is how the trick is done.

But the materialistic worldview, the money and power that is the core of the industrial world, is what the problem is really about. It is time for us all to wake up and take a deep look at our values of life. What do we believe in: Love or money? You cannot serve two masters. You got to choose. The pharmaceutical industry has obviously made its choice. We have made ours. Now it is your turn. What do you choose?

Chapter 7

THE COST OF A PATIENT CURED WITH BIOMEDICINE COMPARED TO THE ORIGINAL, HIPPOCRATIC, HOLISTIC MEDICINE

One of the largest and most burdensome posts on the Danish national budget has been the rising cost of biomedicine. Every year for several decades the cost of biomedicine has risen with 15-20% and it seems that this development continues (182). Hundred of new drugs, often much more expensive than the older, reaches the market every year, and there seems to be no limit for the expenses the politicians are willing to pay for the biomedicine, to keep the people satisfied.

The price for medicine is negotiated every year or so in secret negotiations between the government and the pharmaceutical industry. In Denmark, where we have *socialized medicine*, we often end up paying much more for the pharmaceutical drugs than other countries. It seems that the Danish government and the pharmaceutical industry are best friends. Every economist seems to agree that this development will bankrupt the state in like 10 years if it continues but nobody seems to bother. Least of all the politicians.

How come this blind confidence in the pharmaceutical industry? How come this firm belief that society at large are benefitting from all these new drugs? The pharmaceutical industry has come to have an extremely strong position in the Danish society because of the system of *socialized medicine*. How can it be OK with the politicians that the majority of the tax money in the future is transferred directly to Big Pharma? Don't politicians read science? Don't they notice that in practically all the independent researchers' metaanalyses the drugs don't keep the promises – that most often the drugs simply don't work to any clinically significant degree? Don't the politicians understand the basic principle of *bias*? Well, obviously not.

People not so popular in the pharmaceutical industry, like holistic medical researchers and therapists, are often bothered and "investigated" by the national health agencies, often directly on the initiative of biomedical doctors, most often psychiatrists, who most obviously are serving the pharmaceutical industries interests (70). It seems that the pharmaceutical companies have become so influential that they can make even the national health organs serve its interests, and not the interests of society or the interests of the patients', they were established to look after. Below (Chapter 9) we shall see that the Danish National Medicines Agency is following the pharmaceutical industry almost blindly.

This is truly a scary development. Big Pharma even uses the national health agencies to discipline the doctors that won't push its drugs. It looks a bit like the formula: "Big Pharma + The authority of the national state = Big brother", doesn't it?

The English Cochrane researcher Tom Jefferson gave us an example of the political power of the pharmaceutical industry (215): Imagine that a government would want to remove the cancer chemotherapy from the market (as we shall see in Chapter 8 there might be very scientific reasons for doing this). What would happen? The cancer specialists making research in the new drugs together with the pharmaceutical industry would immediately go to the media and tell "the people" that "Health Minister X is planning to deprave the cancer patients of their life saving chemo cure! He is going to kill the cancer patients we could have saved with this treatment! And this just to save money!" The good story in the media will be to scandalize the politicians; this always sells newspapers.

So who would you believe, if you got the story from the media, *the brave doctors striving to save the patients lives* or *the dirty politicians trying to save some tax-money*? you who are reading this book are smart enough to understand the phenomenon of bias. But when more naïve people than you realize that the persons to be killed (!) next by the politicians most likely is their own mother (!!) and sister (!!!), would they then vote for Minister X or the political party he represents at the next election?

This is the kind of power the pharmaceutical industry has today. It can take a whole government down. It can destroy any researcher that comes in its way with unwanted research. It can even get newspaper journalists fired if they are investigating things about the pharmaceutical industry that should not be known publicly (215). In our capitalistic world money is power and a company worth hundreds of billions of dollars it simply immensely powerful. it is.

The pharmaceutical industry uses its power to make more money. Making money is its *reason d'être*. So what should it do with its money and power if not making more money and getting more power?

In this chapter we investigate how much health we get for all the money we use to buy biomedicine in Denmark. And compare it to the health per dollar we get from buying the classical, psychosocial, Hippocratic biomedicine.

We have already published this analysis based on the assumption that the RCT was valid (165). We have been thorough and made it for all clinical conditions. So we can let you know the result of our analysis right away: The money going to biomedicine is not creating much value. It's simply vast of good money.

We will in this chapter first look at these calculations. In the end of this chapter we will discuss how the same cost-benefit analysis looks if the RCT is not valid. Interestingly it does not make much of a difference. With or without the acceptance of the RCT procedure, money that should buy health is obviously wasted on biomedical dugs.

Cost-Benefit Analysis of Biomedicine: The Cost of a Cure

In Denmark we are about 5 million citizens. The users of the Danish *socialized medicine* are primarily the 2,500,000 chronically ill patients[2]. Half of these are physically ill, half mentally ill. Most of the physically ill patients have severe mental problems, and most of the mentally ill patients have severe physical problems. Both groups have severe social, existential and sexual problems. Half of the chronic patients are unable to work or study normally. Most of people not being ill still have existential and sexual problems. This is the paradox of the Danish society: Almost everybody is rich and satisfied with own life and society at large, and almost everybody is at the same time suffering. Quality of life is rated high on measures that are superficial like immediate subjective wellbeing (42,43) but significantly lower on measures connected to love, quality of relations, meaning of life, sexual satisfaction, and sense of coherence (42,43,230-235).

The total cost of treating the over two million chronically ill patients is above 50 billion DKR or about 8 billion USD a year. As only half the chronically ill patients make extensive use of the health care system, the cost pr. patient can be calculated to about 40.000 DKR or 7,000 USD a year. As these patients often get ill when they are still young and after this make use of the health care system every single year for the rest of their life, the life-time cost for 35 years of biomedical treatment can be roughly calculated as 35x 40.000 DKR = 1,400,000 DKR or 200.000 USD.

We saw in Chapter 7 that if we accept the documentation based on the RCTs only one in a hundred of the chronically ill patient actually gets help. As most of these patients are treated with drugs in Denmark with an NNH=3 we know that about 33 of hundred patients is harmed every years.

As we have seen the RCTs are not to be trusted, so we know that the NNT number is likely to be much higher, and the NNH number likely to be much lower. NNT=1000 is a realistic guess, if the drugs helps at all. And NNH=1 or 2 is a realistic guess regarding the number of patients harmed. Basically nobody is helped and everybody harmed.

This does not mean that there isn't a large number of acute patients with syphilis, boreliosis, meningitis etc. that actually benefit from the treatment with drugs. We are sure there is. But what we focus on here are the many millions of chronic patients that never are cured. These are the vast majority of patients, and the major part of the money to healthcare in Denmark goes to the treatment of these patients.

When we talk about the price of biomedicine this is where the money goes. To treat a syphilis patient from syphilis takes a simple test and a package of penicillin. It is about 200 UDS. Other acute infections cost about the same; a little more if hospitalization is necessary for a few days. Acute medicine is cheap, inexpensive, affordable. It is the treatment of chronic patient that cost real money.

In 2009, strongly inspired by a paper in JAMA (123), our international group of researchers published the first comparative cost benefit analysis, comparing the cost per cured patient with biomedicine and non-drug medicine:

> "*Results*: We found CAM to be 100 (10-500) times as cost-effective as pharmaceutical drugs for most clinical condition. The 50 years estimated cost for one patient cured was for: drugs 1,000,000€; physical therapy 100,000€; psychotherapy 200,000€; mind-body medicine 100,000€; holistic mind-body medicine 30,000€; one-session shamanistic healing with hallucinogenic drugs 2,000€. A large number of clinical conditions could be cured with CAM but not with drugs, which mainly only reduced symptoms. CAM is more efficient than drugs and has no side (adverse) effects and events, whereas treatment with drugs almost always has many often severe adverse effects and events." [165]

In this study we used the data coming from the pharmaceutical industry's own documentation of the drug efficacy and harmfulness based on the RCTs. We found that holistic non-drug medicine was more efficient, much less dangerous, and at least 100 times cheaper per cured patient than biomedicine.

Now, if this analysis is repeated based on the position that results from the RCTs are not to be trusted, how would the results then be? Basically, the price per cured patients with pharmaceutical drugs will rise from 1,000,000€ to 10,000,000€ or 100,000,000€. The whole thing turns into a joke. We are paying billions of dollars for nothing. We are being cheated, robed, deceived.

We conclude as follows in the abstract:

> "*Interpretation*: Drugs turn patients into chronic patients instead of curing. Half the population of the western world today is chronically ill, seemingly because of national health organ's preference of biomedicine instead of CAM. The shift from drugs to CAM would improve health radically in the society and reduce the cost of healthcare to a small fraction…"[165]

We do not know if our analysis has any effect on the health politicians of the world. We say basically that we have the wrong medicine in Denmark, as biomedicine is curing almost nobody and costing an immense amount of money. We could buy so much more health if we went back to the classical holistic medicine. But, if you were health politician, who would you believe? Some crazy holistic doctors doing research that shows that biomedicine is a scamp, or these nice and properly dressed gentlemen from the industry, having fine academic titles and obviously a powerful position in the world, ensuring you that pharmaceutical research has provided the world with so much new knowledge and so many new drugs, so NOW we can help the suffering, sick people of the world TOGETHER?

If you are a smart politician you would think: Aha, the industry is biased pro the drugs and the holistic medical researchers are bias pro holistic medicine, so I will believe none of them. But there is a tiny little difference. The industry is going for the money. There really is no money in holistic medicine in Denmark, where this kind of medicine is not subsidies by the government. We can't be motivated by the money as we are not making any, and as there is no chance in a thousand that we will be rich.

We have collected about 40,000,000 DKR or 6,200,000 USD for our research the last 20 years or so, being the most successful fundraisers ever in the area of holistic medicine in Scandinavia. We have invested every penny received from the research foundations in the research projects. We have not filled our own pockets. We could have done that. But we are not going after the money. We want to change the world. Because the world needs so badly to change.

WHICH TYPE OF MEDICINE IS HELPING THE MOST AND HARMING THE LEAST?

The calculation of the comparative cost-benefit analysis presented above is based on layers and layers of data. It is very easy to manipulate such a calculation by estimating things differently. As we are in an area where little research has been done many figures are estimated, sometimes by other researchers where we have accepted their estimates, or by researchers in our group.

To make the situation completely transparent for everybody we have decided to give all the basic information that our calculations are based on in this chapter. We are sorry if you are bored by this; if you are you are most welcome to jump to the next chapter. But we owe to give this information for the skeptical reader to make up his or her own mind.

The first analysis we give is the simple NNT-analysis for the different kinds of medicine that has been researched. We have included the references to give the reader an understanding of the number of papers every bit of information is built on. In spite of the impressive first look of the tables we need to warn our reader about the fact that most researchers in holistic medicine has not published robust statistics documenting the healing in a way so it is easy to see the NNT numbers (dichotomized data with the outcome cured/not cured).

The way we have approached this problem is basically to see if the NNTs could be fairly estimated from the published papers; if not we have visited the researches, interviewed them about their results, and published the interviews as a supplement to their own work. About half the data comes from the latter approach, making these prone to bias, as we subconsciously, in spite of our best efforts to be objective and neutral, wanted their results to be good. We are convinced that even the most skeptical of researchers will still find similar results, although the results may differ with a factor 2,4 or even 10 because of bias (67).

The source of the NNT numbers for biomedicine comes from the pharmaceutical industry (79). They are likely to be biased also. We know that NNT for most pharmaceutical drugs is about 20 (5-50) (79). This means that between 2 and 20% of the patients are helped with biomedical drugs. These drugs normally only blocks symptoms, and only temporarily; normally they don't cure the patient (165).

Table 1 (165). NNT and NNH numbers of the seven CAM classes estimated from clinical studies (with chronic patients, see text) (based on 39-74, see 17). (see 165 for the references)

CAM class	Short term effect (0-6 month)	Long term effect (6-24 month)	Side effects/ adverse events
	NNT	NNT	NNH
Class 0-Biomedicine	5-50	5-100	1-5
Class 1-CAM (Chemical CAM)	≥10	≥20	25 (allergy)
Class 2-CAM (Physical therapy)	2-4	6	>64,000
Class 3-CAM (Psychotherapy)	3	6	>64,000
Class 4-CAM (Spiritual therapy)	10	20	>64,000
Class 5-CAM (Mind-Body medicine)	2	4	>64,000
Class 6-CAM (Holistic medicine)	2	1-2*	>64,000
Class 7-CAM (Shamanism w. drugs)	1	1	>1000

*The effect of clinical holistic medicine and similar medical systems seem to continue to increase though time (53).

NNT: Number [of patients] Needed to Treat (to benefit) [one patient]. NNH: Number [of patients] Needed (to treat) to Harm [one patient].

Table 1 shows the efficacy for biomedical drugs and the different types of CAM/holistic medicine when treating chronic patients for the first time (second time these patients might be less responsive). This definition is a little tricky for when do we know that a patient is chronic? Presumably, in countries with socialized medicine, first after noticing that the patients are not getting any better when treated with drugs. The NNT number for long-term effect in Table 1 is therefore likely to fit reality more than the NNT numbers for short-term effect.

NNT is number of patients needed for one to be cured (or, for biomedicine, one to be better), and NNH is the number of patients needed for one to be harmed. Mind-body medicine is talk-touch therapy in general. Holistic medicine is focused on the whole person (body, mind, spirit and heart) and is aimed at personal development and self-exploration to gain self-insight and existential healing (salutogenesis) "(155,156). Shamanism has the same goal but uses strong active placebo drugs (hallucinogenic drugs) to induce a powerful, healing crisis often called "metamorphosis" (or adult, human metamorphosis) (100). Researchers in consciousness like Grof and Grof, Feuerstein, and Wilber have often found that this dramatic healing process also can be induced without drugs (24,100,208,295-298). We have seen the same in our own clinic, often leading to dramatic improvement of health in a very short period of time (sometimes a few days) (100).

The general Number Needed to Harm of biomedicine is about 3 (80,110,111,165); for the active placebo drugs used by shamans, the hallucinogens, it is at least 1000 (122). This gives us an idea of the toxicity of the normal, chemical medicine approved through the RCT-procedure. Chemical medicine is in general 333 times as dangerous as LSD. If we go to CAM, we have the types of CAM using scents, flowers, herbs (170) etc. and continued exposition to these items seems to provoke allergy in one in 25. The non-drug CAM therapy can be divided in the high-energy manipulation systems like chiropractic, which sometimes have adverse effects (tissue damage) (not included in the table) and the low-energy manipulation systems like massage therapy, body psychotherapy, reflexology etc which are found to be extremely safe (NNH>64.000) (80,109,111,122).

You simply cannot harm people just by talking and touching them if the patient has agreed to the treatment after full informed consent, if you come from good intention, and if you don't use force. This does not mean that you as a CAM therapist cannot do anything wrong; you most definitely can (30). These errors will hinder or slow down progress of therapy, but they will, according to the statistics, not lead to harm of the patient. But the patient not being helped, as we have seen much too often in CAM therapy, is bad enough.

The CAM types 1-4 in Table 1 are the most popular types of CAM; as you can see the average NNT of these methods are about 6, meaning that 5 out of 6 patients is not benefitting from the CAM therapy. The patients that are helped are rarely cured so in many ways these methods are also only symptomatic, and after a year we have estimated the NNT>10, basically meaning that your chances of real progress using these CAM methods are not very good.

The CAM methods that work are addressing your whole existence (CAM class 5-7). Homeopathy (CAM class 5) works wonders but only if the physician understands the process of healing, in spite of the homeopathic drugs being nothing more than placebo pills in our humble opinion. And often the results are not lasting.

To get a high likelihood of lasting results you need to work directly with the patients philosophy of life, which is happening in classical, Hippocratic holistic medicine (CAM class

6) and in shamanism (CAM class 7). Unfortunately we do not have any data on the success rate of classical allopathic medicine, inducing the healing crisis with toxic drugs. No doubt that the NNH was low, presumably 1; but it is also likely that NNT was high, presumably 1 also.

As the shamanistic medicine men and the classical Hippocratic doctors seem to be equally efficient with the Hippocratic doctors avoiding the adverse effects of the drugs, the classical Hippocratic medicine, that has been the standard medicine in Europe for more than 2300 years, still seem to be most efficient and safest type of medicine. This is why we have chosen to focus our medical research on this kind of medicine (15,37-39).

To understand the intensive use among young people in the western world, where millions use the strong, active placebo drugs – "Acid" (LSD), "E", "Ecstasy" (MDMA), "Magic Mushrooms" (psilocybin, muscimol) etc – it is important to understand that about a quarter of young people have very serious existential problems (42,43).

The active placebo drugs are not magic in a religious sense; they simply allow the user to explore reality on a deeper level and change some fundamental opinions about self, life and the surrounding world from negative to positive (171-174). As our personal reality to a large extent is a materialization of our consciousness and attitudes (17,111), changing these fundamental negative believes will improve quality of life, and thereby also health (111).

It is therefore most likely that the active placebo drugs are helping its users more than they harm, even if they are used without competent guidance by the classical shaman. Most interestingly the DJs often play the role of the shaman in the clubbing environments where hundreds or thousands of young people are taking these drugs together. We do never encourage people to use these drugs, but we must conclude that they have been banned for no scientific reason at all.

We believe the healing potential of love and care to be much larger than the healing potential of the active placebo drugs and we therefore recommend, based on Table 1, the classical, holistic medicine to the patients.

If people want to know more about the principles of shamanistic healing these are many relevant books on these mattes (175-177) and there is a whole tradition of "magic literature" (177-181) that helps the reader realize the basic principles of changing ones personal reality from negative to positive, and one's life from despair and meaninglessness to happiness and the sense of coherence. We recommend all our patients to read Saint-Exupérys book about *The Little Prince* (181) at the beginning of the treatment with holistic medicine in our Research Clinic for Holistic Medicine and Sexology in Copenhagen.

If you can enter this magic universe you can make any change in your life happen. This is why this book has been sold in millions of copies and been translated to almost all languages on the planet. Isn't that amazing? If you are a little smarter you can read Huxley's great book "The perennial philosophy". Huxley explains here basically the same ideas of life and personal development, as Saint-Exupéry. If you are more hardcore you will read the I Ching (179), if you are religious you will read the Koran, the Bible, texts on the Kabala, or the Tibetan Book of Dead (180) ; if you are even smarter you might read Schopenhauer (299). The massage is basically the same in all these books, philosophical and religious systems: Your consciousness creates your reality; only if you love your life will be good. This is also what we found to be true scientifically (17).

Quality of life and health can be improved it you understand you life better, make better use of your talents and becomes more valuable to the world. This is the message of the

Corpus Hippocraticum (3). And today's medical science tells us in line with this that *quality of life is the best medicine* (111).

If you are happy and feel good, don't worry about your health. You will be fine in the future (74-77). Do you need to take vitamins to stay healthy? Most definitely not. No independent, scientific metaanalyses have ever to our knowledge documented a positive effect on health of multi-vitamin pills. If you *feel* fine, you *are* fine. Eat whatever you like; this is statistically connected most with happiness and health (42,43). Don't you worry about a thing! Do you need to take fish-oil in tablets and capsules of herbs to stay healthy? Definitely not! Why would you? What should that help? That kind of CAM (CAM class 1 in Table 1) has never been documented to be very helpful. Don't worry. Be happy. The body will take care of itself if you are. Isn't that magic!

THE LONG TERM CONSEQUENCES OF THE DIFFERENT KINDS OF MEDICINE

In our paper where we published our comparative cost-benefit analysis of biomedicine and CAM, we wanted to see what happened though time with the patients that were treated with the different kinds of medicine. We started by making Table 2, based on the most simple assumption: That biomedicine and CAM was ass efficient in helping patients year 2,3,4, and 5, as they were year. According to this table all kinds of medicine would eventually cure all patients. We know this not to be true in practice, and we learned that medicine obviously is much less effective year one than year two.

The problem here was that the data was of very low quality; both the clinical trials from the pharmaceutical industry and from the holistic medical researchers did rarely run for longer than a year or so; some of the CAM trials ran for a couple of years, but after then everything where in the dark. Instead of using data from clinical studies we approached the problem from a different angle, considering the whole development of medicine in Denmark to be a large scale biomedical experiment. Forty years ago or so we got socialized medicine and ever since the Danish patients has been offers free biomedical care. Instead of this leading to everybody being healthy it has been a disaster for health of the Danish population with every second citizen being chronically ill and permanently taking the pharmaceutical drugs (2,182). Every year more and more drugs are entering the market, but the population health continues to go down (2). From this huge-scale Danish experiment we can learn how biomedicine takes care of a population. The research design here is the cohort study, and as we include all Danes using the great national statistics, believed to be of the best quality on the planet, we have knowledge about the long term effect (40 years) of biomedicine on a very large population of people (5 million Danes).

We do not have data on CAM of a similar quality as CAM has only been popular in Denmark recently (160). The eastern countries that primarily use CAM, like Bhutan, have very poor health statistics. So we don't know much about how holistic medicine keeps a population healthy, but the clinical data from the CAM and holistic medicine studies seems to be better than the biomedical trials, and the outcome is often cured or not cured. In this research (15) the patients experience of his/her health is normalized or not evaluated by use of a measure for self-rated health, which is know the most robust health care outcome of all (73-

78). We have been fortunate that the structure of data is so that we can interpolate the development in patient's health though time from these studies (165). The clinical studies use self evaluated health, the strongest known predictors of the patients' future health, which also to some extent allows us to predict the patients' future health (73-78). All in all we have in this way been able to construct Table 2 to our own satisfaction (165).

Table 3, based on the abovementioned facts, shows that only a small fraction of the patients actually get cured with biomedicine. After 40 years 80% or so of the ill patients are still ill in spite of continuous treatment with biomedicine; if we look at the adverse effects (not listed in the table) we are pretty sure that all patients after 40 years have been harmed. Biomedicine cannot keep a population healthy, as we know, but harm almost everybody in the long run.

Chemical CAM is even worse. Nobody is really helped in the long run, according to our estimate based on research published in BMJ on this kind of medicine (170). On the other hand there are extremely efficient types of CAM like sexology where almost everybody is cured during the first year of treatment; and these results seem to be permanent (240). Such data makes it very easy to predict the future for these patients: They will be good. Classical holistic medicine is not that efficient, as only one in two are cured the first year, but follow up studies have shown these patients to continue their existential healing in the years to come, rather surprisingly increasing health after therapy (201); if therapy continued this result is most likely to even be better. Therefore we can predict the future health of this group of patients also. A lot of clinical research has been done in physical therapy (300), psychotherapy (301-303), and mind body medicine (123-128), giving us a fair basis to guess the future health of patients attending these systems (165).

Biomedicine is much more costly than CAM; it uses a lot of technology that request the patient to stay for extended time at the hospital; CAM is normally done in an ambulatory, also when the most intensive methods are used.

Table 2 (165). The fraction of ill patients cured for drugs and non-drug medicine, if NNTs could simply be added, and health accumulative

Number Needed to Treat (NNT)	Not cured (years of treatment)					
	0	1	2	3	4	5
Biomedicine						
5 (most effective drugs)	100.0	80.0	64.0	51.2	41.0	32.8
10 (typical drug)	100.0	90.0	81.0	72.9	65.6	59.0
20 (typical drug)	100.0	95.0	90.3	85.7	81.5	77.4
50 (cancer chemotherapy, antipsychotic drugs ("mental state"))	100.0	98.0	96.0	94.1	92.2	90.4
100 (less effective drugs)	100.0	99.0	98.0	97.1	96.1	95.2
CAM						
1 (like sexology)	100.0	7.0	0.5	0.3	0.0	0.0
2 (typical mind-body medicine)	100.0	50.0	25.0	12.5	6.3	3.1
3 (typical non-drug CAM)	100.0	67.0	44.9	30.1	20.2	13.5
5 (less effective CAM)	100.0	80.0	64.0	51.2	41.0	32.8

In our estimated of the price of biomedicine above we included the cost to hospitals. One could argue that this is not giving a fair estimate as the hospitals are used for much more than biomedical treatment, i.e. surgery, labor, and hospice functions for the dying. To make a fairer estimate we have excluded the hospital and administrative costs of the Danish health care system and focused on the price of the pharmaceutical drugs themselves using the national statistics (182). From this source and the number of chronic patients in Denmark we have estimated a mean cost for the pharmaceutical products per patient per year of 15,000 DKR (2,000 EURO/2,200 USD). This cost is pretty much the same as the price of one year of CAM or holistic medicine (20 sessions of one hour).

Table 3. Accumulated number of patients cured through time under continued treatment (year one, two, ten and forty) with biomedicine and the seven CAM classes estimated from clinical studies with chronic patients and the state of health of the Danish population after 40 years of free biomedicine (based on 39-74, see 17) (see text) (see 165 for the references)

Class	Fraction of patients cured (percent)			
	First year	Second year	Year 10	Year 40
Class 0-Biomedicine	10	25	20	20
Class 1-CAM (Chemical CAM)	< 10	< 10	< 10	< 10
Class 2-CAM (Physical therapy)	33	50	60	60
Class 3-CAM (Psychotherapy)	33	50	60	60
Class 4-CAM (Spiritual therapy)	10	15	20	20
Class 5-CAM (Mind-Body medicine)	50	75	80	80
Class 6-CAM (Holistic medicine)	50	85	90	90
Class 7-CAM (Shamanism w. drugs)	90	90	90	90

Table 4 (165). Accumulated cost for one patient cured through time (year one, two, ten and fifty) for biomedicine (calculated for NNT = 10) and the seven CAM classes (NNT = 1-10) based on clinical studies with chronic patients (based on 39-74, see 17, and Table 4)[1]

Treatment	Accumulated cost (€)			
	per patient	per cured patient		
	First year	Second year	Year 10	Year 50
Constantly treated w. biomedicine				
Class 1-CAM (Chemical CAM)	>20,000	>40,000	> 200,000	> 1,000,000
Constantly treated w. CAM				
Class 2-CAM (Physical therapy)	4,000	6,000	24,000	100,000
Class 3-CAM (Psychotherapy)	6,000	10,000	46,000	200,000
Class 4-CAM (Spiritual therapy)	20,000	38,000	180,000	800,000
Class 5-CAM (Mind-Body medicine)	4,000	6,000	16,000	100,000
Class 6-CAM (Holistic medicine)	4,000	5,000	10,000	30,000
Class 7-CAM (Shamanism w. drugs)	500	600	800	2,000

[1](cost of biomedical examination, hospitalization, and treatment of adverse effects and events not included) (estimated round numbers, see text)

Table 5 (165) lists the efficacy of CAM for the different clinical condition: Physical health problems, mental health problems, existential, psychological, sexual, and work/study related problems as it is known from the scientific sources. About half of the scientific references are work done by our own international group of researchers. We like to worn the reader about a possible bias from us doing so much of the documentation on CAM, but our results are not differing from the results of the other CAM researchers (see 165). So we are hardly more biased than other CAM researchers, like the physicians Dean Ornish and David Spiegel, psychoanalysts like Harold Searles, or the famous sexologists Masters and Johnson (240).

Based on these data we have constructed Table 4, showing the cost per cured patients with the different types of medicine. As we have set all treatments to cost 2200 USD a year, the variance in price simply comes from the variance in efficacy though time.

Table 5. Estimated NNT-numbers of the CAM treatments of physical, mental, existential and sexual health issues and working disability (mostly based on clinical studies using chronic patients as their own control, see text) (based on 17) (see 165 for the references)

Treatment	NNT	References
CAM for physical health		
Subjectively poor physical health	3	(7-10,13,17-23,39,46,59)
Coronary heart disease	2-4	(71,72)
Cancer (QOL, survival, pain)	2,7,3	(73,74,82,83-88)
Chronic pain	2-3	(14,17,20-22,33,39,46,49,51,54,59,82)
CAM for mental health		
Subjectively poor mental health	2-3	(7-13,17-22,40,50,55,64-66)
Schizophrenia	3-5	(9,11,21-23,40,52,64-66,89)
Borderline	3	(9,11,21-23,40,52,64-66,76,89)
Major depression	2-3	(6-10,20-23,35,40,50,57,64-66)
Anorexia Nervosa	3	(6,20-22,40,41,42,43,64-66)
Anxiety	3	(7-10,12,13,17-22,40,57,64-66)
Social phobia	3	(7-10,13,17-22,40,57,64-66)
CAM for sexual dysfunctions		
Subjectively poor sexual functioning	2	(16-22,41,46,47,51,55,61,62,64-70)
Male erectile dysfunction	2	(41,68)
Female orgasmic dysfunction	1	(41,68,69)
Female lack of desire	2	(16-22,41,46,47,51,55,61,62,64-70)
Female dyspareunia	2	(41,46,47,51,55,61,62,64-70)
Vaginismus	2	(41,46,47,51,55,61,62,64-70)
Vulvodynia	2	(41,46,47,51,55,61,62,64-70)
CAM for psychological and existential problems		
Subjectively poor quality of life	2	(7-10,12,13,17-22,42,47,51,57,64-66,73,74,85)
Sense of coherence	2-3	(7-10,12,13,17-22,42,47,51,57,64-66,73,74,85)
Suicidal prevention (with decisions)	1	(18,19,20)
Low self esteem	2	(6,20-22,43,64-66)
CAM for low working ability		
Subjectively poor working ability	2	(20-22,60)

If you just treat a patient 50 years in a row, with a treatment cost of 15,000 Dkr (2,200 USD) per year this sums up to 750,000 Dkr (110.000 USD). How much it costs to cure a patient depends on how long time each patient on average must go into therapy to get well. With biomedicine only 20% of patients becomes healthy, despite 50 years of treatment. This can be converted to a patient on average must go into treatment in 250 years to be cured with chemical medicine.

Table 6. Estimated first year treatment cost per cured patient with physical, mental, existential and sexual health issues and working disability (mostly based on clinical studies using chronic patients as their own control, see text). As many patients not cured will die it is often difficult to make the long term estimates (based on table 4 and (17) (see 165 for the references)

Treatment	Cost per cured patient €	
	CAM	Biomedicine
CAM for physical health		
Subjectively poor physical health	6,000	200,000
Coronary heart disease	4,000-8,000	1,000,000
Cancer (QOL, survival, pain)	4,000;14,000	20,000,000
Chronic pain	4,000-6,000	500,000
CAM for mental health		
Subjectively poor mental health	4,000-6,000	200,000
Schizophrenia	6,000-10,000	20,000,000*
Major depression	4,000-6,000	200,000
Anorexia Nervosa	6,000	100,000
Anxiety	6,000	100,000
Social phobia	6,000	100,000
CAM for sexual dysfunctions		
Subjectively poor sexual functioning	4,000	no cure
Male erectile dysfunction	4,000	20,000
Female orgasmic dysfunction	2,000	no cure
Female lack of desire	4,000	no cure
Female dyspareunia	4,000	no cure
Vaginismus	4,000	no cure
Vulvodynia	4,000	no cure
Infertility	12,000	20,000
CAM for psychological and existential problems	4,000	no cure
Subjectively poor quality of life	4,000-6000	no cure
Sense of coherence	4,000	no cure
Suicidal prevention (with decisions)	2,000	no cure
Low self esteem	4,000	no cure
CAM for low working ability		
Subjectively poor working ability	4,000	no cure

* no antipsychotic drug cures schizophrenia, and the mental state of patients are in general no improved but hallucinogenic behaviour is reduced (NNT = 4) (75) *(see* 165 *for the references).*

With holistic medicine, the corresponding number, since about 85% of patients are healed in two years, is two to three years. Because there are some patients who are not becoming healthy and thus continues in holistic therapy for the rest of their life, the price for holistic medicine is still rather high. Most patients can be treated for a low price but some are very expensive but much fewer that with biomedicine. Again, the table shows that the Native Americans and other pre-modern people have a radically more cost-effective treatment system than we have in the Western world, using the classical, holistic medical methods.

Table 6 shows atoning differences in the cost per cured patient. Health cost 15-100 times as much if you use biomedicine that if you use CAM, independent of what disease or health problem we look at. Some diseases like cancer and schizophrenia, that almost never are cured with biomedicine makes the cost per cured patient in these groups explode into astronomic figures. Here the value created per dollar is more than 1000 times as big if you buy CAM instead of biomedicine.

Are these figures to be trusted? Well, they are all based on estimates. This means that they might be a factor 2, 4 or 10 different if another group of researchers made the estimations and calculations. So they are not rock solid in that sense. But we find the figures solid in the sense that the figures are in the correct order of magnitude. Curing a schizophrenic patient with antipsychotic drugs could cost 2,000,000 €, 20,000, € or even 200,000,000€. But it is highly unlikely that it can be done for 200,000€.

Doing the same with holistic medicine might cost 1,000€ or 10,000€; it might even cost 100,000€. But it will never cost 1,000,000€, because this would translate into 10,000 hours of therapy. Searles used 900 hours of psychotherapy (mean) and cured one schizophrenic in three (58). We did the same for two patients in only 60 and 100 hours respectively using the tools of classical, Hippocratic holistic medicine (costing 6,000 resp. 10,000 USD) (200). So we have done our homework. We know it can be done from our clinical practice. We also know the amount of resources it takes. Thus we believe our figures to be correct.

We also found (Table 6) that holistic medicine can be used to treat almost all diseases, while many health problems did not have a chemical product intended to cure them.

WHAT NOW WHEN THE RCT IS NOT VALID?

Now, all these analyses are built on the assumption that the RCT is documenting the drugs positive and negative effects correctly. Which we know it is not. Therefore the situation is even worse than that illustrated by these tables. In reality we do not have any scientific reasons to believe that the NNT numbers of the drugs are 5-50, in spite of all the pharmaceutical documentation stating that. It is much more likely that the drugs don't work at all and that all these drug-trials must be seen as commercials for the products, not as science at all. Just looking at bias Gøtzsche found this to be the case for the drugs he examined, the painkillers, as mentioned above (67). But he still found the RCT in itself to be scientific, as he did not consider the problem of active placebo at that time (67).

But the RCT test being invalid really turns the whole thing up and down. We are most likely not to get health at all from most pharmaceutical drug treatments. The pharmaceutical companies have cheated us; the pharmaceutical industry has manipulated the drug-test so it can get lots and lots of poisonous drugs approved as medicine. The Danish society is bleeding money and the health of the population is just going down, down and again down. Everybody is getting poisoned. This really has to stop now.

What are the consequences of using all the money on biomedical drugs?

Basically the money we pay to Big Pharma goes to manipulate and deceive the world yet more. The money could be used better.

The money could obviously be used to improve population health if it bought holistic medicine to the people instead of drugs. We have seen the statistics of how this could improve everybody's health. The money could buy preventive medicine, giving all children and teenagers a thorough education in how to improve their quality of life, how to stay healthy and avoid sexually transmitted diseases and HIV, traffic accidents etc. Large positive youth development programs have been developed in Hong Kong that could be further developed to great benefit of the world (304).

But maybe the money could be used even better yet. We are living on a planet that is burning. A planet that is melting down. A planet with a wild population growth rate, over populating the planet and making too many people destroying too much irreplaceable nature.

Maybe the billions and billions of dollars spent on useless and poisonous biomedicine today – all the money that Big Pharma manage to get out of its grand deception of the world – should be used to save the world. We are empowering a most evil, blind, materialistic and deceptive pharmaceutical industry that obviously only wants to make money, while it falsely proclaims that its intentions are to help and cure – an industry that is manipulating a whole world to believe that it creates value while it does not.

We have been so blind. It is time to wake up and take responsible care of our vulnerable, precious blue planet. Please help us make a better world. Please help us make everybody wake up and understand what is happening. The future of the planet is at stake. We are dead serious about this.

Let's use our wealth to make a better world and make the planet a place where our children can live, survive and be happy.

The most sad thing is that biomedicine keep the mislead people happy with their politicians. The dimensions of the fraud can first be fully comprehended when the political dimensions of this is also taken into consideration. The politicians want to win. That's their game. It's not about doing good, as less as the pharmaceutical industry is about doing well. Politics is about power. Not about love. You can only win if you can pretend that. And if you want power you are most likely also a person that believes in medical science, in the value of the RCT and in the pharmaceutical industries products. So you want the state to buy these products for everybody! These great chemical products that really can improve health! As we have seen in Denmark! Right? It's a joke. Everything becomes turned upside down. The world is fast asleep, while the pharmaceutical industry runs the show.

But don't believe in the nice stories you hear about Denmark and its wonderful system of socialized medicine. It's a lie. It's not true. The Danes are sick. Half the Danes are chronically ill, and they never become better, in spite of free biomedical care – all the drugs in the world. Drugs will make you neither healthy nor happy. Only wisdom and self-insight can do that.

Chapter 8

THE CHEMICAL MEDICINE'S EFFICACY IN THE SERIOUS DISEASES. SOMATIC MEDICINE: CANCER AND CORONARY HEART DISEASE. PSYCHIATRY: DEPRESSION AND SCHIZOPHRENIA

In this chapter we shall look at the documentation of the efficacy of the chemical medicine with the two most serious physical diseases, cancer and coronary heart diseases, and the two most serious mental diseases, schizophrenia and depression.

These diseases are extremely common in the western world; one in two will die from a bad heart, one in three will die from cancer; one on two or so will suffer from depression at one point in time and in spite of schizophrenia only hiding about 1% of the population, schizotypical personality disturbances hit around 20% of the population; and schizophrenia and the more severe personality disturbances are often invalidating disorders that take the often young patient's life down for good unless cured.

About half the beds in all mental institutions are filled with schizophrenic patients. The mental disorders, like schizophrenia and depression, are not diseases in the sense that you either have them or not, as these disturbances come in a spectrum of being more or less schizoid and more or less affectively out of balance. Of course you can define a threshold and say, that if you are so silly or so down, you are schizophrenic or depressed. Cancer is better defined biological, because it can be found in histological tests (histology = science of tissues). In cancer the cells grow and divide wildly and make tumors that spread. The coronary heart disease is also well defined in specific narrowing of the coronary arteries due to break down of the fine structure of the arterial walls.

Mental disorders are about your mind; physical disorders are about your body; statistically both are strongly connected, and both diseases are closely connected to emotional and spiritual health, especially the dimensions of *sense of coherence*, *quality of life*, and *sexual satisfaction*. Most researchers in psychosocial medicine believe that if you have a good life, a satisfying sex life and a good sense of coherence with inner and outer reality, then you will stay healthy till you die. Have great fun in life and stay healthy. If you waste your time your life will be short and your health poor. If you suck you die. To improve the patient's quality of life by helping him or her to make better use of life and talents is the secret of holistic medicine. This was basically what Hippocrates discovered 2400 years ago. And this secret has been known in all pre-modern cultures. Only we, the proud western civilization, do not know it. The reason we don't know it anymore is that there is money in making us believe that we are dependent on drugs, biomedical doctors, high tech hospitals, medical science etc. While these things can be practical for some individuals sometimes, the culture as such are suffering tremendous from the industrial misguidance that removes us from truths.

Throughout this book we have been telling you that biomedicine rarely can provide drugs that benefit patients with severe physical or mental disorders. We have been telling you that even if you accepted the documentation that comes from the RCTs, huge metaanalyses made by researchers at well respected and internationally acknowledged research centers independent of the pharmaceutical industry have systematically documented that the chemical medicine have never been able to cure any patient with one of these four diseases. The drugs don't work. The manufacturers want you to believe that they do; they might even believe that themselves. But better research that the industry can provide has documented that the majority of the drugs prescribed for these severe disorders don't help. They don't cure. Many of them don't even block or hide symptoms. They only poison and harm.

We have argued that while the commercial pharmaceutical companies have every reason in the world to bias their results – billions of dollars, punds and EUROs are to be made if just the numbers come our right – the independent researchers are serving the patients interests, not the industries. Therefore these independent analyses are much more trustworthy that the pharmaceutical industry's RCT-documentation, that for researchers in RTC-bias look more like commercials than as science (67). Thousands of medical doctors are now engaging in the Cochrane movement and tens of thousands of independent metaanalyses are produced to document the true results of the drug trials with the RCT method. The sad thing is that this precious knowledge is not being used. The pharmaceutical world just continues as if nothing has happened.

It is a weird thing about the RCTs that these procedures are so complex and many-layered that you have so many opportunities to intrude a bias, that you little by little through the analysis, by hundreds of small twists get the whole thing manipulated into serious errors. The independent analyses we are going to present results from are more than just independent studies; they are also metaanalysis, meaning that they take the data from tens or often hundreds of single industrial RCT-trials and calculate the results from the original data produced by these industrial trials. The calculations and interpretations follow quite rigid routines (306-308) making it very difficult for the researcher to induce bias and very easy for other researchers to control the quality of the analysis.

Finally the researchers often communicate directly with the researchers who made the original studies to collect also unpublished data from unpublished and published RTCs. The pharmaceutical industry often only publishes the data in favor of their drug while negative research that could harm the companies' economical interests is often not published (67). This is called *publication bias*. If there exist data from other studies like the Cochrane metaanalysis such data must be included in the drug trials; this is almost never done as the Cochrane metaanalyses pretty much would determine the outcome because of the number of studies it is built on. To exclude such studies are called *reference bias*; reference bias is normal in industrial drug trial; to ignore that other researchers have found the drugs or the class of drugs that you are testing not useful is an extremely serious way of cheating the world (67). There should be laws against it. Seriously, there should be.

The lack of personal interest, the rigid protocols, the collection also of unpublished data, the inclusion of hundreds of different studies etc. gives us good reason to trust the results of the independent researchers' metaanalyses and the lack of these things and the many irregular things going on here give us reason to distrust the documentation coming from the pharmaceutical industry (67).

We have in chapter 2-5 documented that the RCTs are not scientifically valid. In this chapter we are looking into another reason to stop accepting the RCTs as basis of scientific documentation: It is so easy to manipulate this complex procedure, and so hard to find all the hundreds of small biases that sums up to major errors, that results from the RCT-procedure are not reliable at all.

Then, why should you trust us, when we bring you these general interpretations of the situation around the RCTs? We have no financial or other interest in introducing a bias. It is more the other way round: The more we give you conclusions that go against the interests of the pharmaceutical industry and the belief of the academic ivory tower of medicine, the more we are likely to get into trouble.

> JM to SV: If we publish this book we will need to wear a bullet proof jacket...
>
> SV to JM: I don't think they are going to kill us. If we succeed in getting this book out, we will be too famous to be killed. It's more likely that we will be discredited and publically accused of pedophilia or of being responsible for some patients' death!

So why do we tell you this? Because we know it. You most likely don't. We are the researchers, and we know. It is out obligation to let you know also. This is not funny. This is very serious. Most of the seriously ill patients of this world are getting the wrong treatment, a treatment that only makes things worse.

There seems to be a much more effective and safe ways to treat patients but you are not supposed to know that. We will tell you so that you will know.

If this book hits the market you are likely to hear all kind of bad things about us. We are fairly old people now and we have never had problems with the police. We have never broken the laws. We have never done any patient any harm. Just don't believe what they are going to tell you about us.

In this chapter we focused on the four most serious and most common diseases that exist; we know that you are about 90% certain to get one of them in your life time. When you do you are in serious need of a good doctor and efficient healing. So you need to know what we are telling you in this chapter. We are telling you what kind of medicine that is likely to help you and what kind of medicine that probably won't work.

We are not referring much to our own analysis of anti-psychotic drugs (81) and anti-cancer chemotherapy (86). Not because we don't find our own work of high quality because we do. But because we know that you will think that we might have biased our own analysis. So we are primarily referring to other researchers analyses. Well, let's just mention here that we found the same as the other researchers. Some of the original analyses were a little old, like Abel's, so we had to check be certain that things had not changed radically since then 1992. It had not. So we simply did our homework to check if these independent researchers had been correct in their analyses, and if it still was so. And they had. And it was.

All the research we will go through in this book accepts the RCTs, which we as you have noticed in the previous chapters have found not to be scientifically valid. But as most physicians and medical scientists do accept the RCT procedure we simply calculated the total risk (NNH_{total}) for a user of the pharmaceutical drugs and compared them to the documented benefits, and we could document that more people were harmed than benefitted. Regarding the drugs used to treat psychosis, all the anti-psychotic drugs, we found that every single patient is likely to be harmed from every antipsychotic drug and no patient at all is likely to get an improved mental health with any such drug, when compared to placebo (81). But this is not new; it has been shown already (133). Nobody seems to care. At least not the pharmaceutical industry and the psychiatrists using their drugs. But now let's concentrate on the four diseases, one by one.

CORONARY HEART DISEASE

Being the primary cause of death in the western world, this is a disease that has been subject to intensive research. But still today there is no drug that can prevent this disease to appear and there are no drugs that can cure it when it happens. There are drugs for the acute treatment that can help dissolve a blood clot that blocks a coronary artery in the hyper-acute phase, but the stenoses cannot be removed by any chemical medicine. These narrowings are caused by a disturbance in the way the cells grow in the vessel and science knows of no drug that can recreate biological order in the body. For theoretical reasons such a drug cannot be found either (91).

Most interestingly there are highly efficient holistic medical cures, the most famous developed by the Californian physician Dr. Dean Ornish (118,119). He has published the great results of his cure that *opens the heart physically, emotionally and spiritually*, in the Lancet in 1990, and in JAMA in 1998, and since then he has been an icon for the international movement of holistic medicine. And sadly also a target for all kinds of attack from the biomedical doctors.

We saw Dr. Ornish give a lecture about his research in California around 1997, seven years after his scientific break-through in the Lancet; he almost cried on the stage sharing his problems with his biomedical colleagues that seemingly did whatever they could to take him down.

His methods are extremely efficient according to the statistics; one in two or three of the patients are radically improved just in 6 months (118,119). The patients come to him with extreme chest pains and without the ability to climb stairs, and after three months these pains has often disappeared.

This is truly amazing. So much heart surgery can be spared, so much suffering. If only the patients knew how bad their prognosis are with the heart surgery and how good their prognosis would be with holistic medicine. About half the patients getting extensive coronary vessel surgery are dead after five years, while only a small fraction the patients are dead after five years if they use Dean Ornish' method.

The problem here is that if you believe in emotional and existential problems as the cause of the disease you will go for a psychosocial cure; if you believe in mechanical causes like bad DNA and unhealthy food, you are likely to go for the surgery and drugs. The patients believing in psychosocial causes would benefit little from a mechanical solution, while the patients believing in mechanical causes presumably would benefit little from a psychosocial cure. Or so we think today; little research has been done to examine the possibility to cure non-believers with holistic methods. The opposite have been tried many times and it does not work. We think that people not understanding the principles of psychosocial medicine could learn these principles as they are fairly scientific, and this would make psychosocial medicine work for many of these patients… It would help a lot if the country's national health agencies would recommend a psychosocial treatment and not only drugs...

So it ends up like always being a question of politics and money. There are big money in heart surgery, and small money in supporting the patients' self-exploration and teaching the patients love, intimacy, self-esteem, sexual freedom, and integrity. So Ornish has to fight for his institute's life. The Lancet paper helped him of course. So did the JAMA paper. But these papers also started an evil campaign to take him down. This campaign has been so successful that today, 20 years after Ornish brilliant research break through, his methods are hardly in use at any hospital in the western world (except in Ornish's own hospital in California). All the patients are still getting heart surgery, in spite of the rather poor destiny associated with the surgical treatment, and the great prospects with holistic medicine.

Dean Ornish success with holistic treatment of coronary heart disease is an outstanding example of the healing power of classical holistic medicine compared to biomedicine – both drugs and surgery included. And the political problems Dr. Ornish is facing are so typical for doctors who choose to use love and compassion to help their patients heal, instead of surgery and drugs.

We need the politicians to start taking these things seriously, and make laws that protect the holistic physicians and holistic medical researchers and empower the patients to choose the treatment they like freely, and not influenced by biomedical propaganda and political pressure from the strong lobbyism of the pharmaceutical industry.

Every second person living in the western world will die from a bad heart. So you might be happy to know that holistic medicine can in fact prevent a bad heart. Just stay happy and in close connection with other people and your heart is not likely to fail you. This was what we essentially learned from Ornish studies. If you heart fails you, it is not too late to learn to love. Just start today and you heart will most likely heal. Isn't that beautiful?

CANCER

One in three citizens gets cancer in the western world. This is a gold mine. A diamond mine. A money tree for the pharmaceutical industry and the doctors using its products. An anti-cancer treatment often costs a hundred thousand dollars or more. So if you divide the number of patients in the western world, divide it with three and multiple it with 100.000 USD, you see the economical dimension of this. It's about 3.000.000.000:3x100.000 USD=100,000,000.000.000 USD in the bank, just waiting to get paid out. Well, we think most people will agree that this is good money. It's what we call *a fine business opportunity*.

No wonder the pharmaceutical industry has been digging into this goldmine for years. The big thing is anti-cancer chemotherapy: Extremely poisonous drugs (like mustard gas used as a war gas during world war II) that *in vitro* – in the lab - seems to kill dividing cells more aggressively than none-dividing cells. As cancer cells are rapidly dividing, the rationale is that the cancer cells are more sensitive for chemotherapy than the rest of the body's tissues.

Most unfortunately are there so many fast dividing cell types in the body that this nice idea isn't based on much biological reality.

As you can imagine there has been so many randomised trials of chemotherapy for so many different kinds of cancer that you simply drown in studies. As you might expect, if you understand how the RCT procedure works, most of the published, industrial randomised clinical trials (RCTs) have documented a positive effect of these extremely poisonous drugs on quality of life and survival.

With our present knowledge of the extreme toxicity of the drugs, and of how the documentation from RCTs can be biased and manipulated, and most often are, combined with our understanding of the extremely strong financial motivation for creating such positive documentation, is it only a natural thing to be a little skeptical about the pharmaceutical industry's positive results.

An independent research center in Germany decided about 1985 to collect all data on the treatment with chemotherapy of the most common cancers, called the epitheloid cancers: Cancer of the lung (small-cell), lung (non-small cell), colon/rectum, stomach, pancreas, bladder, breast, ovary, cervix, uteri, and endometrium.

The researcher who collected the data for the largest and most thorough cancer metaanalysis the world have seen till this day was the acknowledged German statistician Ulrich Abel. Abel wrote to more than one hundred cancer researchers and asked for all their original data, published as unpublished.

Abel successfully collected almost all relevant data from all studies worldwide through a continued effort that lasted until 1992. He used this unique database to analyze the effects of anti-cancer chemotherapy for all the common cancer types, in five different ways (82); he also published his data and all calculations in several books (83-85). Table 1A and 1B below are his original tables from his scientific paper published in 1992 (82).

We have, in the end of table 1B counted the number of positive (+) and negative (-) findings regarding the effects of chemotherapy for the different kinds of cancer (86). As Table 1A and 1B show there is no tendency to increased survival or improved quality of life for treatment of any cancer with chemotherapy. Abel found quite on the contrary that cancer chemotherapy almost always destroyed the patient's quality of life and shortened his life. Chemotherapy kills you. It ruins your happiness and wellbeing. That was Abel's conclusion. He put that kindly in his abstract (82). But reading his text you cannot be mistaken about this: Abel found that all the drugs used for cancer chemotherapy are strong poisons with no positive effects at all. Well, if you have lung cancer you might die two months later (mean) according to the RCTs. But you will die and the quality of the rest of your life will be significantly worse if you choose to take chemotherapy.

As you might expect the reaction from the pharmaceutical industry was extremely negative towards Abel. All kinds of negative rumors were started and he was discredited in many different ways. In the end he was forced to abandon his research in cancer chemotherapy. He told us that the research center's computer broke down short time after his publishing of the data and that the institute lost all the data he had spend years on collecting - and that his back up also disappeared at the same time. Somebody did not like his research. And somebody did what they could to stop it. And somebody succeeded. But Abel's meta-analysis still exists. And will continue to exist. The loss of all data means that his analysis cannot be repeated. They can be reconstructed from the tables in his books though. But why shouldn't we trust Abel's analysis?

Strangely enough his important paper is almost never cited in newer papers on cancer chemotherapy. This kind of bias in research is as mentioned above called *reference bias* (67) and is well known from research in industrial biases. On study that analyzed this problem found that 41 out of 111 pharmaceutical drug trial reports, or 36,9%, had reference bias, and in the large industrial studies with many references, it was 23 out of 33, or 69.7% (305).

This is not good. It is most definitely cheating just to omit the data you don't like. This is the key characteristic of the science done by Big Pharma. These people should not be allowed to make science. They can obviously not manage the responsibility.

If you badly want to market chemotherapy, and live to make money, why would you give a reference to a large metaanalysis that without any doubt has documented that it doesn't work? And risk that some national agency reads it and refuse to approve your drug? And loose a billion dollars. That would be kind of stupid, wouldn't it?

So what has happened is that the pharmaceutical industry and the cancer doctors first discredited Abel and after this the industry simply has chosen to ignore his important work. But Abel's metaanalysis is still the leading star in the dark about the effects of chemotherapy. And since the data has been destroyed, and the pharmaceutical industry has stopped testing against *no treatment* no more scientists will analyze this. Ever. Smart move, Big Pharma.

But this does not mean that the cancer drug industry did not learn from Abel's study. It became evident that whenever you randomize to *no treatment* as was done in most of the RCTs used in Abel's study, no treatment would be better for the patients than cancer chemotherapy - if you avoided *bias in data analysis*, meaning that if you just calculated the statistics correctly.

It can hardly come as a surprise that "A statistician who wishes to favour one drug over another has many options" (67). But it is really sad that it makes so much of a difference who is analyzing the data, the pharmaceutical industry itself, or a neutral statistician. Just a simple recalculation makes about 10% of all the significant results from the pharmaceutical industry insignificant (6%, 8% and 15% respectively in three studies, see review in (67)), and the author concluded that in all the drug trial reports he studied "all errors favoured the new drug." (67) This means that the industrial researchers simply made up the results. They seemingly just filled the results into the results tables so the results fitted their company's needs. When the calculations showed something else they changed the results so they could get the drug that was not working even in their own RCT studies, approved by the national authorities.

Do you realize the consequences of this? The pharmaceutical industry took in about 10% of the drug trials – obviously consciously as all errors was in the industry's favour - poisonous drugs, which from the industry's own drug trials and statistical calculations had no beneficial effect at all, and made it look like the drug were beneficial, simply by "fixing" the tables. As the drugs looked effective they were later approved and sold to innocent patients, who with a little help from their doctor naively believed in the information on the drug label, so the company could make even more money.

So it is no surprise that Abel's study has been ignored in spite of the fact that the abstract of Abel's paper can be found in www.pubmed.gov, which is the large database of medicine, where every medical researcher on the planet starts to look for scientific documentation.

The pharmaceutical cancer drug industry started after 1992 to make the RCTs with the new drugs against the old ones. This was smart, , because if you just made the poison stronger in the new drugs than in the older (or increased the doze), and measured over sufficiently short time, and with the "optimal" local (non-global) outcomes, as we have seen, the active placebo effect would be on your side and you would win.

So since 1992 there has been hundreds of cancer chemotherapy RCTs involving hundreds of thousands of cancer patients, who most likely all have been harmed, and who most likely did not benefit at all, in spite of a similar number of RCT-based industrial papers documenting the positive and excellent development of the cancer chemotherapy treatments.

We made our own metaanalysis of all cancer RCTs with cancer against *no treatment* (we took these data from over 100 Cochrane metaanalysis of cancer chemotherapy giving you an idea about the magnitude of this branch of research) (86) and found, in spite of a much more limited body of data than Abel had, about the same result as Abel did 17 years earlier (82). We included all types of cancers, not only the epitheloid cancers as Abel had focused on. We found, if we used the data from the RCTs that chemotherapy a least for some cancer types could prolong life for a few months but that it statistically could not safe any lives. As it ruins your quality of life and does not make any significant clinical difference to survival, it is not worth it. As the choice of chemotherapy is likely to exclude a choice of holistic medical treatment that might help at least some cancer patients, as we have seen in the previous Chapter 7, your choice of chemotherapy seems to be the wrong choice if you want to survive your cancer.

Abel found, still accepting the data from the RCTs as valid, that chemotherapy does not help patients with the following type of cancers: Cancer of the lung (small-cell), lung (non-small cell), colon/rectum, stomach, pancreas, bladder, breast, ovary, cervix, uteri, and endometrium.

We basically found the same for all types of cancers in general, in a study that also respected the validity of the RCTs. There might still be some cancers in children that can be cured with drugs; our study cannot exclude that possibility. But we can conclude that in general, cancer chemotherapy is extremely poisonous; statistically it will harm you, ruin your quality of life, and it will also kill you. Statistically you will live shorter if you have one of the above mentioned types of cancer and you choose chemotherapy (82).

According to our analysis presented in chapter 1-5 of this books the documentation based on the RCT-method is not scientifically valid. We also know from Abel's metaanalysis that all these scientifically looking documentations from the industrial anti-cancer chemotherapy trials filled with data on improved survival and quality of life are not to be trusted. If you accept that the RCT method is not scientific and the results from this method are not valid, the results of chemotherapy on cancer patients are likely to be even worse than Abel found.

There is no doubt in our minds that the pharmaceutical cancer drug industry should have been shut down after Abel's results in 1992. This did not happen; the pharmaceutical cancer industry was much too powerful. And now every biomedical cancer researcher in the world tries to ignore Abel's work and forget about his results. This is a scandal. Hundreds of thousands of patients suffering from a "experimental" treatment that we already know is bad.

Cheating, cheating, cheating. If you say it the right way, you can make it sound much like a cash register. Katjing katjing katjing. This is how it works. You manipulate the world, and make a billion dollars, and the whole world will bow to you honor. You screw and poison every helpless cancer patient, and steal their money, and everybody will pay you respect. This seems to be the most problematic aspect of the capitalistic world. We don't say that a Maxistic-Leninistic world is any better… we don't think there is an alternative to capitalism. But if we are not aware capitalism is as much about power as other political systems: it is all the same dark, political materialism. The antidote to this is awareness, consciousness, understanding. We desperately need a new world order, based on consciousness, love, and ethics, to save the future of the planet and to make people living today happy.

Good medicine is about love. This is how it has been for more than two millennia in Europe, ever since Hippocrates. Good medicine is not about manipulating the world to believe that extremely poisonous drugs can be helpful, so that you can sell them to doctors and patients just to make money.

Think about it for a moment. You have presumably also believed in cancer chemotherapy at some point in time, maybe till this day. We hope that you find the documentation we are provided convincing; we think it is. And it this is so: How could you ever be fooled into believing that strong poisons could help a sick person? What happened to your common sense? These drugs were used as chemical weapons during world war two, and now you think injecting mustard gas should be good for your body? Sorry, no offence intended, but where did you park your brain?

THE SHADOW OF OUR CULTURE

In our modern society we believe so much in science that we are willing to repress our instincts and feelings and our common sense. But when we wake up, we go: "Oh yes, I knew that all the time… I felt it in my stomach, something was not right…" We just did not want to use precious life energy on these stupid matters. It is difficult to believe in something else than most people. It is painful to wake up. It really is. Because then you are alone.

But we think that we and everybody else has an obligation to seek, find and share the truth. Only in this way can we help the world to grow and develop. It needs our continued effort every single day to correct all the lies and manipulated truths we meet that rise from all kinds of personal interests. We must fight all these lies. We must be awake an aware. Else we simply fall prey to the dark, commercial powers of the modern capitalistic world. The shadow of our culture.

The big pharmaceutical companies are behaving just like predators. As are the biggest and smartest of these other big companies in the weapons industry, the tobacco industry, the chemical industry etc. They eat people for lunch. They don't care about human lives. They don't care about the global eco-system. About pollution, deforestation, explosive growth rates, and planetary destruction. If you suffer, even if you die, this doesn't matter, as long as they make money. And they do. Big money. Colossal money. Incomprehensibly large amounts of money. Money enough to buy the whole world. Which is what they do these decades.

THE ROLE OF WHO – WHAT DID WE LEARN FROM THE SWINE FLU SCANDAL?

How much money did the Swine Flu vaccine companies make? How dangerous was the swine flu compared to normal influenza? What was the role of WHO in the marketing? What are the relations between WHO and Big Pharma then? Did the vaccine have any adverse effects? Did it harm more than it benefitted? Who are the true winners when the whole world is fooled to buy billions of doses of unnecessary and also harmful vaccine, as the vaccine has adverse effects as all other pharmaceutical drugs, for tens of billions of dollars? See? They eat you for lunch.

Table Ia. Direct evidence from randomized studies on the question of whether palliative chemotherapy prolongs survival. (Ø: There is no evidence of this type. + or ÷: The evidence is definitely a positive/negative response. (+) or (÷): Unclear evidence; on the whole rather positive/ negative. In case of (+) and (÷): the effect is, if any, small.)

Type of study:	Site Chemotherapy + X vs. X alone (X = any treatment)	Immediate vs. deferred therapy	Dose-effect studies
Lung, small-cell	+	Ø	÷
Lung, non-small cell	(+)	÷	Ø
Colon/rectum	Ø	Unclear	Ø
Stomach	÷	Ø	Ø
Pancreas	÷	Ø	Ø
Bladder	Ø	Ø	Ø
Breast	÷	(÷)	÷
Ovary	Ø	Ø	Unclear
Cervix Uteri	Ø	Ø	÷
Endometrium	Ø	Ø	Ø

[Our explanation to the analysis: First study series is Chemotherapy and any other treatment vs. this treatment alone. Second study series contains trials with immediate vs. late, deferred chemotherapy. Third study series is dose effect studies, where the efficacy of different doses of chemo therapy is tested, from very low to very high].

Table Ib. Indirect evidence on the question of whether palliative chemotherapy prolongs survival. (Ø: There is no evidence of this type. + or ÷: The evidence is definitely a positive/negative response. (+) or (÷): Unclear evidence; on the whole rather positive/ negative. In case of (+) and (÷): the effect is, if any, small

Type of study:	Site Randomized comparisons of different regimens	Non-randomised comparisons of patient cohorts	All 5 measures - [our conclusion]
Lung, small-cell	+	÷	+ + ÷ ÷
Lung, non-small cell	Unclear	÷	(+) ÷ ÷
Colon/rectum	÷	÷	÷ ÷
Stomach	÷	÷	÷ ÷ ÷
Pancreas	÷	÷	÷ ÷ ÷
Bladder	÷	÷	÷ ÷
Breast	(÷)	÷	÷ ÷ ÷ (÷)(÷)
Ovary	+	÷	+ ÷
Cervix Uteri	÷	÷	÷ ÷ ÷
Endometrium	÷	÷	÷ ÷

[Our explanation to study series 4: Documentation collected from randomised comparisons of different regimens; fifth study is evidence from non-randomized patient-cohort studies. Last column is the results from all these five types of evidence taken all together].

WHO is reported to have made a strong alliance with the Influenza Vaccine Industry (309); to sell the vaccine the fear of Swine Flu was boosted internationally though the media, and it was "predicted" that "1.8 million people would need hospitalization and 300,000 would end up in the intensive care units (ICU). Further, they predicted that hospitals would be overwhelmed and that ICU units would not have enough beds to care for the sick and dying. Incredibly, they predicted that 90,000 people would die."

In the end it turned out that the Swine Flu was almost harmless, much less harmful than the normal flu. What happened was that WHO had been taken by Big Pharma and use for marketing purposes. It is as ugly as it can be. Scare everybody to buy unnecessary, harmful drugs! That's how to make money. How do we stop this madness? Well, now we have written this book, and if you also do something, and other people also help bring things back in balance, we will eventually.

CAM IN CANCER

One argument often heard by people defending the pharmacological cancer drug industry is, that there are no alternatives to chemotherapy. But there obviously are. One alternative is no chemotherapy. Just to refuse. And to use the money to find some nice people to care for you. To do this makes a lot of sense, especially when it comes to patients with one of the cancer types that Abel found were not helped at all by chemotherapy. So this is one possibility: Just don't take it. Refuse. Say no.

Cancer is very hard, challenging, and troublesome indeed. But don't accept to be abused also. You don't have to suffer more than you do already. We don't think you have deserved it. Be kind to yourself. Love yourself. That is the only way. And don't take drugs that have proven to be only poisonous. Don't make it worse. That is the first thing.

But then there are also real alternatives to the biomedical treatment. Holistic medicine has a lot to offer cancer patients. It has been documented that psychosocial treatment can improve quality of life for patients with metastatic cancer (121,187). It was even documented in one study that the patients that improved their quality of life lived twice as long as the patients in the control group (121).

This study was made at Stanford University and published in the Lancet in 1989. Some of these patients, females with metastatic breast cancer, miraculously lived for more than 10 years, while all patients in the control group, that did not improve their quality of life, all were dead after five.

Holistic treatment of metastatic cancer patients has also been seen to induce spontaneous remissions in one patient in seven according to independent and critical analyses (121,185,186). We know that CAM therapists often promise to cure the cancer patients and that they often do not succeed, which is also cheating and deception, . CAM therapists are also human, and they can lie or be mislead by their own success with some patients to believe that they can cure all.

There are many small private cancer CAM hospitals. In Denmark we have Humlegaarden (188), who for years have treated with orthomolecular medicine (claiming to us the "vibrations" of the molecules; we find it to be spiritual medicine, CAM class 4 in Table 1). From the number of successful case stories published at the hospital's home page, and the total number of patients estimated, it seems that one in ten or so of the patients are getting a spontaneous remission here, which is not bad at all. We know that the national Danish health agencies are controlling this website, and comparing every case story published with the patient's case record to be certain that the information is correct (189). This is in accordance with the NNT=10 for spiritual therapy in table 1. The number is estimated from available data; it could be 20 or more. Unfortunately the owner of the hospital as many other CAM therapists does not believe in the value of statistics so he has refused to make the statistics in spite of us asking him for it (189).

We have seen patients with metastatic cancer improve their quality of life and get spontaneous remission in our holistic medical research clinic too. Sometimes these remission were only partly, where the tumors have been reduced in size (190,191), sometimes complete remissions happened where the metastatic cancer disappeared totally and stayed away for years (192). So they are happening, the spontaneous remissions.

The Danish researcher Ulrik Dige found 45 cases of well documented spontaneous remission (245), and interviewed them to understand what had happened before they got their spontaneous remission. It turned out that these miracles were not really spontaneous but happened after the patients reflected deeply on his or her philosophy of life, and improved it by letting go of negative believes. A spiritual awakening had happened in two out of tree cancer patients. The rest found a strong and lasting will to live, like they woke up from a long lasting sleep on a deep existential level. Both groups of patients seemed to take learning from their cancer disease before they were suddenly cured. Which is in line with the classical Hippocratic holistic medicine, as the reader may notice.

To self-exploration, personal development, and improvement of quality of life, guided by a wise, loving and caring therapist will greatly enhance your chances of survival. We recommend the classical talk-touch therapy. Find somebody to love and care, even if you have to pay for it. Anybody will do. Just make sure that the love is genuine.

To conclude this section on cancer, one in three will get cancer. You are likely to get it, but first when you are rather old, don't worry about it. If you have cancer, know that chemotherapy is not very helpful in most cases. The CAM treatments seem to work, but little science exists to tell us what kind of CAM is the best for cancer patients.

We recommend the classical talk-touch therapy as this has helped patients for thousands of years, patients who were likely to also have had cancer. But in reality it is much less about method that it is about personal chemistry. As "the doctor is the tool" (129) in holistic therapy, and love is what makes the magic happen, you'll better find a CAM-therapist or physician you really like (love, adore, or even desire!) and who is able to love you back and genuinely care for you.

According to the statistics we have studied it seem that the best of the CAM therapists can help about one in seven of cancer patients to get a "spontaneous" remission. If you believe firmly in gurus like Sathya Sai Baba (120) the miracle will seemingly happen even more often.

But you need to be your own doctor also. You must start to explore the reasons that you got the cancer in the first place. In this exploration you might find something important you have to learn about life from your disease.

If you are lucky your disease will help you to find new will to live and a brand new understanding of the whole universe (32-35,37-39). If you do it is a very good sign of you finding the inner resources needed to win your battle against the cancer and heal. Alternatively you might find the peace, strength and understanding needed for making the rest of your life a meaningful journey, with little pain and suffering in spite of living permanently with your cancer.

From the statistics it is clear that even with the best of CAM therapy most cancer patients are not cured. But many cancer patients manage to improve their quality of life in holistic therapy (NNT=2). (121,187) These patients simply live a good life, with their cancer reminding them every day of the meaning of life and of the importance of staying on the bright side and of being of value to others. Which is what is really important in life when it comes down to it.

DEPRESSION

Another fine business opportunity is depression. Especially if you can define depression in such a way as almost all patients could benefit from an anti-depressant drug. This was what happened with Fontex and Prozac. For a period of time about 15% of all American citizens were taking Prozac or a similar drug and America was the "Prozac Nation".

Then it was realized that uhhh, maybe there are adverse effects... yes, surprise, surprise. You take a strong poison, a chemical substance that is highly biologically active, transgress the blood-brain barrier, and interacts directly with your brain cells, and rather surprisingly there are adverse effects. What were you thinking?

Antidepressant drugs come in two major classes, the drugs for small depressions and the drugs for major depressions. Recently the effect of all anti-depressive drugs has been studied in details in Cochrane metaanalysis where the focus have been the RCTs where the antidepressant drugs have been tested against active placebo (132). We have mentioned this study in the book already, and we will not repeat ourselves here, but just remind you that the metaanalysis showed, in spite of respecting the validity of the RCT procedure: The antidepressant drugs have no effect at all compared to active placebo.

The result comes from following the Cochrane protocol and removing one study that is highly significant but strangely varying from 7 other studies strongly indicating that something is not right with this study. If you read the paper you will learn that the Cochrane standard protocol requests you to analyze the data for consistency, and if you do that you are obliged to exclude studies that are very different from the rest as these most likely are strongly biased and flawed. When the researchers did that they found that one single study gave all the significance there was, and when they excluded this bad study, all significance were removed from the results.

CAM FOR DEPRESSION

What is depression from a holistic point of view? Depression is not caused by to little serotonin in the brain as the biomedical psychiatrists believe; we have examined that hypothesis and found it not to be scientifically substantiated (101). But what is it then? Well, it's a state where you are overwhelmed by the world and not able to materialize your dreams of creating value and doing good. It's a state of existence where you have lost connection with your purpose of life, your life mission. So the only real source of happiness, which is contributing with your gift to the world in all relations, is out of sight. Therefore, inside of you, there is darkness. You need to reconnect to the life inside of you again, and to the outer world again. You need to get back to your existential roots. That so many people are getting depressed can easily be understood from the unconstructive and doll way we life, the way we abuse our self and let our self down, and the way we are not understand our selves at all. The solution is of course to get a life. To get back in the game. To find somebody to love and spoil, and to learn to receive their love in return. Life is simple. It is always about love.

In this chapter we have learned that antidepressant drugs have no specific, positive, pharmacologic effect at all for patients with depression. In spite of all the physicians and patients believing in them and every day experiencing that they help. But they do. The placebo effect that comes from active placebo is fairly strong. But then, when there are only specific negative effects (harm) from the drugs, why not focus on the consciousness-dimension and use this only, and avoid the poisonous drugs? That was how the old physicians created their marvelous results. These methods are psychotherapy, existential therapy, and holistic therapy and they still exists; they are highly effective for depression as we saw in the previous chapter (NNT=2-3 according to Table 5), and they won't harm you. Much research in psychotherapy have documented the efficacy with depressed patients (NNT=3, NNH>64.000) (80,301-303). As sexuality is important to get the energy moving, it has often been recommend that the therapist be of the opposite sex when treating mental disorders like schizophrenia and depression (54,55,57).

In our own clinical research we found holistic mind-body therapy where the body is also included in the treatment to be about double as efficient as psychotherapy for the mental disorders (NNT=2) (113). So if it is possible for you we recommend skin-to-skin contact to be part of the treatment.

So if you are on these antidepressant drugs we strongly recommend that you skip the drugs and find yourself a nice and competent therapist – and do it today. A Rosen therapist, a gestalt therapist… it doesn't really matter what system you use. What matters is the quality of the therapist. For the doctor is the tool (129).

Is this more expensive? Well, it might be this year, but then again, you might not need to take antidepressant drugs every second year for the rest of your life. That's pretty expensive to. And, you know, if you get adverse effects that might bring you to a hospital as 5-8% of all admissions to hospital departments of internal medicine is due to adverse effects of such drugs (310). This is expensive too. And then you might not be able to work so well. For an extended period of time. This is expensive too. So if you think about it, therapy is not expensive. It is good for you.

When the strong antidepressants tested in the study don't work, there is no reason at all to believe that the mild antidepressant drugs should work. The Cochrane metaanalysis showed that anti-depressive drugs are only poisonous; the seriously flawed RCT-method had made the drugs look like efficient and harmless medicine. But we were tricked.

About 6% of the Danish population and something similar in the rest of the western world are still taking antidepressant drugs (182), in spite of this Cochrane study having been published for years now. And who should stop the pharmaceutical industry from selling these drugs? The national drug-approving agencies should withdraw these drugs now as we know that they only contain poisons.

But again, what would happen if the ministry of health would try to do that? How many hours would it take for stories about patients committing suicide because of lack of these lifesaving drugs etc to hit the front pages of the boulevard press? For how much longer would the minister of health have his chair in the parliament?

What a horrible world of money and political powers and lies and lies and lies. Political power and money is obviously more important than human life. This has to stop. We need a more humane world. And we need it today. Please help us making it come.

SCHIZOPHRENIA AND PSYCHOSIS

The so-called anti-psychotic drugs are used for schizophrenia and psychosis. In chapter 4 we discussed the many different outcomes that are documented in the RCTs testing these drugs.

The drugs are sold as "antipsychotic drugs" but they have no antipsychotic effect. They do not have any beneficial effect on the patient's state of mind according to an large independent Cochrane analysis (133). The outcome related to mental health is called "mental state" and mental state is never improved in the RCTs. We have made our own analysis of the efficacy and harm of the antipsychotic drugs (81), and have found the same. Why nobody seems to care and tell the patients that these drugs do not help them have been a mystery to us.

The sales of antipsychotic drugs in Denmark correspond to 6% of the population taking these drugs every day (182). The yearly turnover of the drugs in Denmark, a small country of only five million citizens, is about a billion DKR or 150.000.000 US$. We estimate the worldwide yearly turnover to be hundred times this, or about 15.000.000.000 USD.

The drugs are strongly sedative and calmed the patients down so they cannot behave badly (81,133) and so they can be talked into obedienc (136). This is highly practical as the psychotic mentally ill patients often are difficult, loud, violent, sexually aggressive etc. What seem to happen is that these patients, instead of getting the therapy that could help and sometimes even cure them (196,200), are just getting drugged down and placed on mental institutions, or if they are not violent and troublesome placed in small apartments in the city under the necessary supervision and "psychiatric care".

My ohh my, is this bad. Hundreds of thousands of young people in the west are given psychiatric diagnosis every year and for the rest of their life they will be chronic mentally ill patients taking the antipsychotic drugs. Instead of having the therapy that could cure at least a large fraction of them.

The adverse effects of the drugs are many and serious, both to the body and to the mind (81,133). Often these people cannot study or work, they cannot get friends and family; they cannot function normally in so many ways that they are severely handicapped. The psychiatrists believe that this is caused by their disease; but we think it is caused by the drugs used in the psychiatric treatment. As the adverse effects impact on quality of life, general ability, and global health has never been documented (as these outcomes are not included in the RCTs) we do not know. But we feel certain that if the drugs had any positive effect in any of these areas, the pharmaceutical industry would have been the first to measure and document it. In the beginning of the RCTs with antipsychotic medicine questionnaire were used that gave a good impression of what happened to the patients quality of life. But these outcomes have been removed. Because the antipsychotic drugs do not improve the quality of life of course.

Patients treated with antipsychotic drugs often commit suicide (210), and we know that 15% of the schizophrenic patients, who are treated with these drugs for many years, commit suicide in the end in Denmark (211). Swedish researchers have suggested that these suicides could be caused by drug induced depression (134). This seems to be a very likely hypothesis. The drugs are extremely poisonous and follow up studies in Denmark by the national health agency has documented that if patients take antipsychotic drugs and other drugs also, their likelihood of spontaneous and unexplainable dead is 50% above normal (209).

How harmful are the antipsychotic drugs? We analyzed this for all types of antipsychotic drugs and found that every single patient that takes an antipsychotic drug is likely to be harmed (NNH_{total}=1) (81). All the antipsychotic drugs were equally bad (133). And equality ineffective in improving the mental health (the mental state) (133).

So what is happening here? Why are these drugs still on the market? Why haven't the national health agencies all over the planet removed these bad drugs from the market? These drugs are obviously the most damaging, harmful, poisonous, killing drugs you can imagine. How can the psychiatrists believe in them when the independent Cochrane researchers conclude that they don't improve the patients mental state?

You can visit mental institutions and see how patients who have taken these drugs for just a few years are becoming. It is horrible beyond belief. When the drugs 50 years ago started to hid the marked the doctors noticed that they did not have to do lobotomia (cutting the Corpus Callosum that is connecting the two halves of the brain to calm the patients down) any more as these drugs had about the same effect (193).

What are we doing to these patients? How can we do that? What are we thinking? This has to stop! Now!

The problem is of course that the biomedical psychiatry has gone so far astray that it is difficult to find the road again. The psychiatrists have been so dependent on the antidepressant and antipsychotic drugs that they cannot any longer treat patients without the drugs.

One of our most important projects these years is the development of contemporary holistic psychiatry; we have now written about 40 papers on holistic psychiatry and related matters and our first textbook on holistic psychiatry is planned to be ready about the same time as this book hits the street (311).

We want to show the psychiatrists and the world that there are other ways to treat the patients than using the drugs, and much more efficient and much less harmful ways.

It is quite understandable that it is difficult for the national drug agencies to remove the psychiatric drugs from the market, because of the strong commercial and political interests in these drugs. It does not make it any easier that the national health agencies often hire psychiatrists as their leaders, employees and consultants.

This makes the whole system very conservative and all administration strongly biased in favor of the psychiatric drugs and of biomedical psychiatry in general. The typical biomedical psychiatrist loves power games of all sorts. They love being part of pharmaceutical industrial research; they love to use force on the patients, they go for the important jobs in the public health system. No wonder the pharmaceutical industry likes them. They are worth every penny.

CAM FOR SCHIZOPHRENIA AND PSYCHOSIS

Schizophrenia and other mental disorders can be successfully treated. Philippe Pinel (1745-1826) had his holistic clinic in Paris about 1850 and he made the first statistics over his success rate with psychosocial medicine for mental disorders; he found that of the many patients who entered his hospital about 70% were cured (197). In the last century many good psychodynamic psychotherapist like Bleuler, Jung, Reich and Searles worked on schizophrenia and the other mental disorders (46-58,194-197).

Harold Searles made an experiment that documented the power of psychotherapy in schizophrenia; he took 18 schizophrenic patients who had been hospitalized for years and gave them 900 hour of psychotherapy each; after the treatment could 33% leave the hospital and live outside; 33% was significantly improved, and 33% were not improved (196). Many such rapports, most with individual patients, have been recorded, so there can be little doubt that psychotherapy and holistic medicine are efficient treatments for schizophrenia (196,197).

Wilhelm Reich insisted on including bodywork in the treatment (55,56), as did the Hippocratic doctors (3). In our Research Clinic for Holistic Medicine and Sexology in Copenhagen we have also treated schizophrenic patients with mind-body therapy, and we have found that these patients often can return to normal function in society after treatment (200). The treatment methods used for this are described in our papers and books on holistic medicine in general (37-39,311,312), and on holistic treatment of mentally ill patients (198-199). We don't think that these methods are complicated or difficult at all; it's just about giving the patient love, care and support to go though his or her own process of existential healing (salutogenesis (155,156)).

We encourage all researchers who want to engage in this exciting endeavor to document the results of treatment by use of the Open source protocol for clinical holistic medicine (15), and we are, as editors of Journal of Alternative Medicine Research, happy to receive your submission of the papers coming from this research (submit to jmerrick@inter.net.il).

Can schizophrenia and these disorders by understood? Oh yes, we think so. And it is not so hard. You need to understand man as consisting of body, mind, spirit and heath. Schizophrenia is the dysfunctional condition that comes when you shut your body and sexuality down, when your feelings freeze because of emotional defenses, when your mind turn the world upside down because of your mental defenses, and your heart closes because of a long history of emotional pain coming from difficult relations with your parents as a child. If you do not know what a psychological defense is you should read some Freud, Jung or Reich, these researchers have explained it very well (53-58).

But the short version is that we need to survive, and often we are not loved the way we are so we have to modify ourselves to be loved by our parents. So we twist our own existence to be loved. Some people twist themselves so much to fit to their parents that when the parents are no longer there they cannot function in the world. The cure is the untwisting. Getting back to your self. Which is what all good therapy is essentially about. If you want to understand this better we are happy to recommend our scientific papers and new book on holistic psychiatry planned to be in the book shops 2010 (311).

CONCLUSION

In this chapter we have look at the efficacy of biomedicine for the two largest and most serious physical diseases, coronary heart disease and cancer, and for the two most serious mental disorder, depression and schizophrenia (including the schizoid personality disturbances).

We have systematically found that there is no biomedical cure for any of these diseases; there are simply no drugs that improve the health of the patients who suffers from one of these four diseases, which eventually will hit about 90% of all people living in the western word.

When you get really ill there is not biomedical cure.

This does not mean that there are no drugs for the patients suffering from these diseases; there are plenty and almost all patients will get these drugs. But the drugs have, according to independent researchers' metaanalyses no positive effect at all; the drugs are just poisonous; they destroy your quality of life and they shorten your life. Statistically they will often seriously harm your mind and body, and they will sometimes even kill you, or make you kill yourself. These drugs are poisons. They are NOT good for you.

Yet these drugs are sold disguised as beneficial medicine because the pharmaceutical industry has managed to develop the randomised clinical trial procedure (the RCT test method) into the perfect tool for making drugs that just are very, very poisonous, into seemingly beneficial and almost harmless chemicals.

We have seen that that in spite of the pharmaceutical industry's intensive efforts to document positive effects of the drugs, the raw data, when these data are analyzed by independent researchers in large metaanalysis, still reveal that the drugs are only poisonous and not beneficial.

So maybe the RCTs are not that good in making poisons into medicine after all. Maybe we are wrong. It might just take a lot of bias, statistical manipulation, manipulations with references, tables, conclusions and abstracts etc. to make the drugs *look* beneficial.

Maybe the whole problem is all about bias, about the pharmaceutical industry introducing bias in favor of the drugs they want to market. If that is the case, no method in the whole world, not even the most rational, can save us from Big Pharma's poisoning of the people of the world, that is if the pharmaceutical companies are allowed to make (or "sponsor" as it is often called) their own drug trials.

Gøtzsche wrote in his doctoral thesis on *Bias in Double-Blind Trials* that "At a consensus conference in 1984, 31 of 36 academics agreed that in an industry sponsored trial, the manufacturer should not perform the final data analysis, whereas only 6 of 46 industrial representatives had the same opinion" (67).

This problem is as old as the pharmacological industry itself. Every sensible person understands that this is not OK, the way these things regarding the chemical medicine are managed in society. But yet the craziness just continues, year after year with more and more drugs hitting the market, and being documented to be bad, and staying on the market. Why is that? Because of the power of the money. If you want to understand what is going on in the world, just *follow the money*.

Who can stop this? Well we can, being doctors, as we chosen not to give our mentally ill patients drugs but use the classical, holistic, psycho-social medicine. Is it easy? No, most definitely not. Well, it is easy to help the patients just by loving them and caring for them. But it is not easy to do this surrounded by critical biomedical colleagues that often behave as if they were sworn enemies of all holistic, psychosocial and alternative medicine.

But as more and more physicians join us, and choose to work with methods that do not harm patients and to not take expensive insurances and equipment, things will be easier. And as more and more patients want this kind of non-drug treatment it will be easier still. And as society at large starts to understand what is happening and politicians start asking critical questions, it will be easier to provide holistic medicine. The solution is in the awakening of the people, the rising of consciousness.

The pharmaceutical industry and the biomedical doctors are often behaving terribly towards people involved in CAM and holistic medicine (70,216). The pharmaceutical industry and its allies, the biomedical physicians, have been extremely aggressive, to protect its own interests, and it has served its own interests in almost any imaginable way. We therefore need strong laws to protect holistic physicians and researchers from the constant evil attacks from the biomedical establishment.

But the government and the national health organs that should make the laws to secure that research in holistic medicine is possible, and that doctors can treat their patients the most efficient and safe ways, are much too busy helping the pharmaceutical industry close holistic medicine down.

Why are the national agencies not interfering when they notice that much stronger and much more trustworthy scientific evidence shows that the drugs don't benefit and only harm? Why don't they withdraw the products from the market when it becomes obvious that the scientific documentation from the pharmaceutical industry is of a much too poor quality? That drugs have been approved that really should not have been?

You probably know the answer already. The whole thing is political. This is why the people appointed directors of national drug agencies are never the cool, good guys, the people who have done independent drug research for many years, but almost always people who have spent years and years doing industrially sponsored research, securing both their solid income and a great academic carrier. Most often these people are devoted drug researches, very often psychiatrists, of course.

So what can we do about it? If you are a patient you can start thinking about what kind of medicine you like. What kind of treatment you need to get better. If you are tempted to take a drug, which you often will be, because of all the golden promises coming from the pharmaceutical drug company who manufactures your pills, and who wrote the drugs magnificent qualities on the label, please think again. If your doctor is insisting on you taking this drug, ask him for a thorough explanation of the drugs function. If this explanation sounds reasonable, if it makes good sense, well, then the drug is most likely OK. You can try it for a period and see if it helps. Make a diary and write down in every detail how you have been the last month. After three month, write again how you have been the last month. And now compare. Are things better for you? Was any improvement because of the drugs or are there other more reasonable explanations (new job, new boyfriend, etc)? It difficult to do. Often it is better to ask a close friend: Did these drugs help me at all, in your experience? If yes, in what way?

If on the other hand, your doctors story is some blurry, smoky talk about some strange things going on in your brain, and he just cannot explain it because “it is very complicated but this is really good science”, don’t believe him, don’t believe a work of what he is saying. If there is a rational mechanism, your doctor will know it, and he will be able to explain it for you. Clearly. Strange medical hypothesis are not a good reason for you to take strong poisons. Even if some drug company, that makes money on their product, recommends it. Or have convinced your doctor. Don’t be a fool. Think!

Chapter 9

THE MARKETING STRATEGY AND THE VALUES OF BIG PHARMA

Recently every second commercial from pharmaceutical companies on TV in Denmark was found to be illegal (313). In itself this is not very remarkable. So many companies are violating rules and regulations. But when you think about it this is a rather high fraction. And you can imagine what their problem with the law is: They are making their products look better and less harmful than they are obliged to do according to the law.

We found this information in the journal of the Danish Medical Association. This journal is careful about not criticizing the pharmaceutical industry without a good reason. So we believe that this information has been carefully checked.

Many pharmaceutical companies do not respect the law when it comes to making money. This seems to be a fact.

BRUTAL, MANIPULATIVE MARKETING CLAIMING: EVERYBODY IS HELPED (AND NOBODY IS HARMED) BY OUR DRUGS!

For 2008 Welt-Online reported that the US pharmaceutical industry spent almost double the amount on advertising (57.7 billion dollars) than it did on research (31.5 billion dollars); but Marc-André Gagnon and Joel Lexchin of York University, Toronto, estimated that the actual expenses for advertising are higher yet, because not all entries are recorded by the research institutions (314). It has thus been estimated that about one third of the total turnover of the pharmaceutical industry is used for direct and indirect marketing. We estimate that a normal user of media in Denmark is hid directly by a commercial for a pharmaceutical product 5 times a day, or 1500 times a year.

Now imagine that half the commercials are illegal and dramatically oversell the drugs. What would the impact be? We guess you would think here: Isn't it enough that they bias their RCTs, that they use the method that over-exaggerate the good sides and eliminates the bad sides of the drugs… do they really have also to violate the law to get their products sold? Well, you see, this is basically about getting their products sold. It obviously doesn't really matter much to many of these companies if it is done legally. Or if the documentation is scientific and trustworthy. Come on now, don't be tense about this. We are here on this planet to have fun, not to be bores.

The typical commercial mentions the positive effects documented in the RTCs in such a way that the most often modest symptom blocking effect on one in twenty patients (NNT=20) is made look like an impressive effect on every single drug user. This is the consequence of using "horizontal risk measures" as we shall discuss below. At the same time the adverse effects are mentioned as little as possible, and often not at all.

The pictures used for the drug commercials are always of normal, healthy, sexy, intelligent, beautiful, young and obviously rich, well-dressed and stylish people who look like the ideal of our culture - very much the same imagery as is used by the tobacco, fashion, car, and female-beauty industries. This way the pharmaceutical creates the idea in everybody's head that the pharmaceutical drugs are harmless, extremely efficient and used by people who are on the top of the world. The message is clear: Be a winner, use our drugs!

We all know that this is not true; it is not the winners that use pharmaceutical drugs (sleeping pills, anti-depressant pills, anti-psychotic pills, pain-killers, anti-anxiety pills, anti cancer drugs etc). Most definitely not. All the good is only happening to the drug users in the commercials.

But the problem is that there are so many layers in these cleverly done commercials. Normal people who consider themselves smart analyze the first or a couple of these layers and think they are not influenced by them. But all the deeper and more profound layers (promising you "mana": power, wealth, beauty, popularity, and sexual potency) will still affect your unconscious mind and make you more positive towards the chemical medicine. Your mind cannot win over perception. It works much like real life experiences.

The many different ways the pharmaceutical industry is using its money to impact the world to buy its products are really impressing. Alone in the USA the pharmaceutical industry has employed 7000 people as lobbyists toward the public USA to promote the biomedicine[216]. Thousands of meetings and congresses for doctors and other medical personnel are sponsored every years, hundred thousands of physicians are paid for participating in research; hundreds of universities are getting founded; and tens of thousands of sexy, goodlooking young girls (often former chearleaders) are visiting the GPs medical clinics every week to tell them about the fabulous effects of the new drugs, showing a little leg and a little breast to make sure that they are also welcome next week. This is so primitive. But it works. Else the girls wouldn't be there. The pharmaceutical industry *understands* marketing. If we generalize the numbers for USA mentioned above, about 300 billion USD is used every year on Big Pharma commercials worldwide. You see, they are good at it. They have experience. They are the professionals. They are better to manipulate us than you might like.

And then there is the "money for research". This sounds very serious, very scientific. Everybody respects that. Money for science. Sounds good. 31.5 billion dollars used in the USA on research budgets. About 150 billion dollars used worldwide (2008, raising about 10% each year). But what is this money really used for? Well, sponsored RCT-studies, with hundreds of thousands of patients, money for researchers and physicians, funding of research cooperation with academic institutions, publication in scientific journals etc. If you look into it, you will see that this budget is not financing rocket science. Because most biomedical drug research is not rocket science. You simply modify a molecule or two in 100 different ways, runs it through a lot of animals to see if some of the new drugs have the wanted qualities, and then you run the pretest and the RCT test on humans. Please. This is not rocket science. This is applied organic chemistry. Not much more than that. We understand that if you know nothing about chemistry this world of chemical labs might be fascinating and extraordinary. We (SV) have spent many years in chemical labs. It is not rocket science to make new drugs. It is easy, it is a simple technique. That is why we have thousands of new drugs entering the market every year without making any difference for the public health (and hundreds of thousands of new drugs being tested on an astronomical amount of animals); meanwhile every second citizen in countries with socialized medicine remains chronically ill[2].

Almost all the medical journals are paid by the pharmaceutical industry in some way or another, giving an almost absurd bias in favour of the drugs; many of the journals are simply not publishing negative results (67),contributing vastly to the major problem of publication bias, as we have seen. The pharmaceutical companies are even financing their own patients' associations indirectly marketing their own drugs while pretending to serve the patients interests.

It is a public secret that Big Pharma has taken over the WHO and other super-national health agencies as discussed above in relation to how successful the Swine Flu vaccine has been sold to whole countries - in spite of the new influenza being much less dangerous than normal influenza, and in spite of the vaccines having so many also quite serious, adverse effects.

The problem here is really the volume of the commercials in the public media and the medical journals, the massive lobbyism, the huge impact on the physicians, the academic institutions and the states agencies that should control and regulate the drugs. Everybody is bought. Everybody is influenced by the propaganda. In Denmark we have documented that the Danish Medicine Agency is not actually controlling the information on the drugs. The information used for national drug directories are provided by the pharmaceutical companies and they are obviously not confronted with the existing information on the drugs and classes of drugs from the independent research like the Cochrane collaborations metaanalyses (315). Basically the pharmaceutical industry dictates what information that gets out the patients and their physicians about the pharmaceutical drugs.

This is really a horrible situation. Who is there now to control the pharmaceutical industry? Who is able to make the neutral and objective analyses of the positive and negative effects, and the evaluation of the total therapeutic value (is it all in all benefitting the patient or is it not?) of the drug? Nobody is, in reality. And this is why the pharmaceutical industry has such an easy game taking over the world. There is nobody to stop it. Nobody to correct it. Big Pharma has grown so big that it has taken over the control of the organs supposed to control it. The state has become the smaller part. Big Pharma wins it all.

Who is the looser when Big Pharma wins in this way? The patients indeed, but not only the patients. We all are. The whole culture is getting shallow. Everybody is getting doped. Mankind is falling to sleep instead of reflecting deeply upon life and disease, and taking learning from the experience of the body and mind not being in balance. Our planet is tilting because we are losing the grip. This is a disaster.

THE PEOPLE OF BIG PHARMA AND THERE LIFE VALUES

Let's start with admitting that we only are medical researchers, and not politicians nor experts in economy. When we in this chapter report on the power of the pharmaceutical industry we are doing it from our perspective as medical researchers. And from our personal experiences with the people from the pharmaceutical industry, and the people who work closely with them.

From our experience with these people from many years or research at the University Hospital in Copenhagen (Rigshospitalet), the prestigious castle on biomedical research in Denmark, we can report on the behaviour and values of these people. We could do research on it but we have decided not to. Life is too short, and we are pretty sure that you will understand the picture, when we tell you about our experiences.

We were both in charge of research in psychosocial medicine at the University Hospital for a number of years. We did psychosocial medical research: research in quality of life and health. For many years (1980-1989 and 1990-1994 respectively) we were leading the research in the famous Copenhagen Prospective Perinatal Cohort at the University Hospital dep. 7112. Since we stopped here we have continued the research from our own independent research institutes.

What we have noticed during these years is that the colleagues that are involved in industrial drug trials are often rich, and that they often make a fine academic carrier. They are often getting all kinds of privileges and they never miss money. They can pretty much do what they like. And they develop an attitude of serving and admiring the pharmaceutical industry. They serve Big Pharma.

We have also noticed that the colleagues working together with the industry almost always are strongly opinionated regarding psychosocial medicine which they normally don't like or believe in.

We have also noticed that these people normally know very little about the more philosophical aspects of natural science, like quantum chemistry, advanced cytology, histology, brain physiology, biological order, evolution, morphology, morphogenesis, molecular self-organization, and the theories for emerging order like the chaos theory, theory of complex patterns, mathematics of complexity etc. They know as little about ecosystems, evolutionary theory, and Gaia theory.

Their primary focuses as biomedical researchers are advanced protein chemistry and regulatory biochemistry. The people of the pharmaceutical industry only know about pharmaceutical drugs and the biological receptors they might interact with. And some related theories. And it seems that they often think this is the whole world, everything there is to know.

It is a religion. Chemistry is their religion. They believe in it.

They are often surprisingly intelligent. They are power players. They know about the power games of the world. They are very political. Good with money. People of smooth character. Eloquent people. They are networking. Helping each other. Throwing good parties, dressed elegantly in smokings and tuxedos.

They are often materialistic people. They like expensive cars, great houses, flashy jewels, expensive red wine and a good steak. They love conferences in exotic places like Hawaii, traveling on business class, and five star hotels. The dress lovely. They like quality. Good smells. Scents, fragrances and perfumes. They are superficial people, with nice facades. They are aesthetic uptown people. They are not only doctors; they are way superior to the average GP. They are the *heroes*. The people that make the world move forwards. They are the MEDICAL RESEARCHERS. You can't get any higher.

People envy them, and wants to be like them. This is why so many young doctors dream of getting access to this wonderland of biomedical research. But only the best are chosen to be researchers, high ranged doctors, professors. The rest will only be GPs, low ranged hospital doctors or administrators.

Researchers have described the medico-industrial complex consisting of the academia, the doctors and the industry, and a large part of the public administration and national health agencies, where these people take their turn on shift, being directors, consultants, highly ranged doctors etc.

Biomedicine is a religion. It is also a community in itself. Lanctôt called it the Medical Mafia[220]. But it's not a mafia in that sense. They normally don't shoot people and they don't have one single boss (or, they may have, but then we don't know him). Every pharmaceutical company behaves as its own clan. And these clans work peacefully together. As the money the industry gets increases every year, everybody is happy. Every clan is doing good.

Almost every pharmaceutical company is making more money every single year. It is more like a community of people who share the same strong belief. They believe in chemical medicine. They pray to it. The protocols for the RCTs are like bibles. Holy books. They worship them. As the content is the same in all the holy books, the holy procedure of RCT, they all share the same religion.

The people of Big Pharma are turned towards the world; they are serving the power structures of the world to benefit from them. They have this nose for power and money; this ambition to be rich and well liked.

The true power of the pharmaceutical industry lies in its willingness to share its wealth and power with all its *friends*. It's very much like Microsoft's strategy of sharing the created value in a pyramid with Bill Gates at the top. In the pharmaceutical industry the money is just so much bigger. Everybody needs a computer software (200US$). But everybody also in the end needs 10 years on Prozac (20,000 US$) and maybe also a cancer chemo "cure" (100,000 US$). See the difference? There are a hundred pyramids or so. And these pyramids are growing every day. Big Pharma grows faster than ever because it has reached a critical mass where its people are everywhere. Its money is everywhere. Big Pharma is everywhere.

IDEOLOGICAL MANIPULATION: CONTROLLING THE RESEARCH

But the indigenous ways of Big Pharme do not stop here. It goes even deeper. Biomedicin – chemical medicine - has its ideology, which states that the DNA-molecule is God-the-creator and that the physical and mental disorders are inherited, and not therefore not curable with psychosocial medicine. Massive research projects have tried – totally unsuccessful in spite of all claims – to document that the human genes are closely linked to diseases like cancer, heart diseases, schizophrenia, depression etc.

The biomedical researchers trying to document the biochemical hypothesis for the diseases has dominated the research the last 30 years, and they have always received great founding and much support, while research projects in psychosocial medicine, holistic medicine, and CAM haven't been supported financially or politically. The biomedical researchers are promoted to professors and placed strategically in the national organs donating money for future research, giving yet another empowerment to biochemical research. The researchers in psychosocial medicine are systematically marginalized.

We have experienced that biomedical researchers from national research centers have called the foundation that supported our research in psychosocial medicine and told them all kinds of horrible stories – unsubstantiated rumors - about us to make these foundations stop funding our research. And about every second time they have tried have these biomedical professors and psychiatrists succeeded with this destructive behaviour.

We have also at several occasions seen the Danish Ministry of Health and other public organs act directly in favour of biomedical research and directly against research in quality of life and holistic medicine. Most people believe the public offices to be objective and neutral, but this is most definite not the case. Nothing is more political than public health research. And nothing seems more controlled and dominated by biomedical and industrial interests.

The sad thing is that in research the results depend on the way you ask. If you ask: Is schizophrenia inheritable? You are most likely to get a yes, if this is the answer you want. This is the basic problem of positivism, as pointed out by Popper.

Even the research questions asked are controlled by Big Pharma. We have often experienced severe pressure to pose our research questions differently; we have been promised money and privileges if we did, and severe problems of all kinds if we did not. You wouldn't believe these things happening in research which is supposed to be objective; but if you think deeper and understand that *belief* is what sells the drugs, not scientific facts (as they in most cases are not convincing enough to make anybody take the drugs) you will realize the importance for the pharmaceutical industry – for the medico industrial complex - of controlling the research.

This basically means that you cannot trust the results of medical science at all. It is totally biased pro biomedicine and drugs. It is done in smart ways so you cannot always see the connections. When massive national programs for healthy food make everybody believe that there should be a strong connection between green low fat high fiber etc diets and health this has never been documented; all these statistic connections between life-style and health are very small compared to the much stronger connections between psychosocial factors like quality of life and health[243]. But as quality of life and psychosocial factors are rarely incorporated in the research, nobody knows that.

Thus the pharmaceutical industry is totally integrated with the academic medicine, the national health agencies, the national research centers, and the physicians and hospitals. The industry is always generous with money and help to its friends. The medico-industrial complex is totally dominating the health sector in all countries with nationalized medicine. Let this be a warning to countries wanting to implement this model. Don't copy the Danish system. Just don't go there. It couldn't resist Big Pharma and now it is corrupt.

WHO PROVIDES THE DATA FOR THE NATIONAL DIRECTORIES OF PHARMACEUTICAL DRUGS?

We will end this chapter with a more technical analysis of the Danish national drug directory. This is the key source to information about the pharmaceutical drugs used by all physicians, pharmacists and patients in Denmark. So if you know who is providing the data for this drug directory, officially based on information on drugs, the drug resumes, from the Danish Medicines Agency, you know who is in power over medicine in Denmark.

We have published an analysis of the product catalog "Medicin.DK" (315,316).

Pharmaceutical product catalogs are large books with thousands of pages every year sent to the medical doctors, clinics, hospitals, libraries, etc. They are normally paid by the pharmaceutical industry. It is made in collaboration between all the parties with interests in the pharmaceutical drugs, like the pharmaceutical industry, the Medical Association, the National Board of Health, etc. As you might expect that the catalog only contains product information from the drug manufacturers and not from the much more critical sources like the many Cochrane studies that often document that the pills do not help much.

At a first glance a pharmaceutical product catalog looks quite scientific. You cannot see the information there is omitted and missing. Only experts can tell what data has been wrongly left out.

We have learned from visiting the Cochrane library that there are thousands of Cochrane metaanalysis now on the effect of the pharmaceutical drugs for many different clinical conditions. When we have gone though the Danish drug directory we have systematically found that the data given here to the physicians and patients are the numbers provided by the pharmaceutical industry itself and not by the Cochrane analysis. Take anti-depressant as an example. The Cochrane metaanalysis found that the anti-depressant drugs do not help the patients; on the other hand they are poisonous and many patients are harmed by them (132). If this information known since 2004 went into the drug directory, all anti-depressive drugs should be removed from the catalog. They aren't. If you are a user you are not even informed about the study – which is reference bias, .

The same goes for all the other drugs we have discussed in this book. The National drug directory ignores systematically all the Cochrane analyses in spite of these studies being high quality meta analysis made by researches independent of the pharmaceutical industry. Made by the bad people. The enimies of Big Pharma. So these studies are simply ignored. Thousands of metaanalyses. Ignored. We therefore know for sure that the data for the Danish drug directory comes from the pharmaceutical industry. That this is a fact has been confirmed by the Danish Medicine Agency itself (315).

VERTICAL OR HORIZONTAL RISK MEASURES?

Pharmaceutical catalogs starts often with a discussion of the different methods for documenting effects (called "risk measures" because we are trying to avoid a risk, typically death). To manipulate the reader the drug directory often uses two different types of endpoints for the positive and the negative outcomes; these types are called “vertical” and “horizontal” risk measures.

A vertical risk measure is something that notes when life, good health etc stops, at a particular time (like a road tree that suddenly stops the traffic); a horizontal risk measure is more like the length of a blind alley, which could be longer or shorter but will eventually stop.

Vertical risk measures (316)

The effect on survival at a given treatment for chronic disease are frequently expressed by means of relative or absolute risk reduction (RRR and ARR respective) or Number Needed to Treat (NNT) / Number Needed to harm, (NNH), representing the “vertical distance between the two survival curves”, measured at an arbitrary time. The distance and the derived measures RRR, ARR, NNT and NNH therefore depend on the measurement date.

Based on the proportion of dead or survivors at any given time the patients of the treatment and control groups are typically measured before the treatment starts and again after 5 years of treatment. (The outcome could be anything but the well-defined outcome “death” is normally used to explain this).

We choose to call these sizes DB (the proportion of deaths in treatment group) and Dk (the proportion of deaths in the control group).

The treatment effect can now be expressed in different ways:

The absolute risk reduction (ARR):	Dk-Db
The relative risk reduction (RRR):	(Dk-Db)/Dk
Number Needed to Treat (NNT):	1/ARR
Relative risk (RR):	Db/Dk
Odds ratio (OR):	(Db/1-Db) / (Dk/1-Dk)

In research with another treatment goal (outcome), such as improvement or healing, NNT and the other risk measures are calculated in exactly the same way. All that matters is that the outcome is dichotomous, so you can say “yes” or “no” to a question about its actual presence.

Horizontal risk measures

In chronic illnesses the efficacy of the intervention can also be expressed as the postponement of time to the adverse event occurs. Each patient is experiencing (in average) that death occurs slightly later than it would otherwise. With this goal, we do not know whether it is one patient in 100 who is lucky enough to get well (one patient wins the lottery) or whether it is all patients live 14 days longer ("small for all").

CRITICISM OF THE NATIONAL MEDICINE DIRECTORIES

It is known from research that patients as well as doctors and politicians rarely prefer a treatment when the treatment effects is measured as NNT (317).

A critique of the NNT measure has been that "neither doctors nor patients can understand it" (316,317). In the pharmaceutical catalog Medicin.DK 2010 (316) it says "Many people also believe that "NNT of 16" means that "15 patients did not benefit from the treatment". This usually mistaken belief is shared by many doctors, according to a Norwegian study (1065 (318))."

It is true that there often are many useful effects of a treatment which is not about the goals you set for it. We thus discovered that many of the patients who were treated for sexual difficulties with vaginal acupressure experienced that their quality of life and mental health were improving as a result of this treatment (about 90% of patients experienced to be helped in one way or another)62. Nevertheless, it would probably not be reasonable to count these benefits as it was sexual problems the patients wanted to be treated for.

We think that the Norwegian doctors have a very different attitude to NNT than the pharmaceutical industry; the conclusion that doctors are not able to understand this very simple endpoint of NNT is not likely to be true. After 7 years at university most people understand the formula: Number Needed to Treat (NNT) = 1/Dk-Db. Most high school students could understand it. This formula is in the curriculum of public schools 6th-9th class, although not everyone learns to divide the number 1 with a difference.

IF YOUR BODY WAS A CAR: NNT AND THE "HORIZONTAL RISK MEASURES" EXPLAINED

Let us try to see a little deeper into what this is really about. Assume for a moment that your body is a car. You have been out in a minor collision and received 20 scratches in the paint. You now proceed to a repair shop and ask them to do your car. If you are told that every second car leaves the workshop in perfect condition this correspond to NNT = 2 for the treatment outcome "perfect health". You would obviously like to know in advance whether it can succeed in making your car, but the damage is so severe, you are told, that it cannot be known in advance. Would you take the chance? We think you would.

If the NNT is 20, this means that you only have 5% chance to get a perfect car back. Would you buy this service? Probably not. Unless you are incredibly happy for your car. Or unless you are satisfied with a worse-than-perfect result.

Here comes the "horizontal" risk assessment into the picture. Now your automobile painter says that "Approximately 50% of scratches disappear on each car. Is this OK for you?" Will you now say: "It's annoying, but OK." Or would you reject the treatment and instead have the whole car side changes? If it is not feasible because you are very poor, you will probably still say yes thank you (provided that no car painters can guarantee you a better result) and find yourself running a battered car. It is after all much nicer than before.

But what if the repair man states that "approximately 5% of the scratches disappear on each car"? It's like every 20 car is perfect, but now this effect is distributed on all the cars ... It is obviously easier to guarantee for the repair man as he do not need to be particularly good. But we doubt that you would say yes to this treatment of your car. You will laugh at the offer and go, would you, shaking your head hundred meters down the road. You will not pay a lot of money for a service that does not make any visible difference.

How does the chemical medicines relate to these statistics? NNT is for most drugs found to be about 20 in the RCTs, we have learned (79). But only very few chronically sick people will get cured by a treatment with pharmacological agents, as we saw in Chapter 6. It is probably only about 1% of the patients that gets significantly better (165). Measured in NNT, this corresponds to a true NNT around 100. Such a NNT will never sell drugs to a patient. If the doctor said: “And one in a hundred patients will be cured, isn’t that amazing!” you would probably say: “What! Is this a lottery?”.

To sell the drugs you are much better helped with the horizontal dimensions that states that “almost all patients are helped (a little). This is good news and most patients will go: “Yes! I will get better! Nice to get this great and promising possibility.“

But what about the adverse effects? The rationale for the whole chemical medicine is that you can get better, but you must accept some side effects. If everyone gets a little better, and everybody gets a little harmed also, it's not likely that somebody will be helped in all, is it?

Therefore the adverse effects are always presented using the horizontal measure (Number Needed to Harm (NNH)). Only one out of 10 gets an adverse effect! Only one out of 20 get seriously harmed! Only one out of 1000 will die! Then all will be helped (horizontal rapport on the positive effects) and only a few will be damaged (vertical rapport of the negative effects). In this way both doctors and patients are mislead by pharmaceutical manufacturers; very few can see through this cunning deception. It is really clever made.

Back to auto painter. There are also side effects of the treatment – dents!. If he tells you that "I can make your car - there is a 50% chance of a perfect result - but unfortunately there is also a small risk that I will make dents in the car, so some 5% (one out of 20) would be returned with a dent.” Now, would you buy this service? Yes, you probably would.

On the other hand, if he said that "there is 5% chance of a perfect result and 5% likelihood of a bump" you would you laugh and say “No thank you. This will lead nowhere.”

But what if the car painter goes: “All the cars I work on is getting better and it is rare (5% of cases) that there will be dents”? This sounds appealing, right? So you go: “Yes, thanks, we have an agreement.”

But what if he said: "All cars are nicer in the paint, and all cars will also get a small dent"? Then you will say no again: “You make some scratches and give me some dents in return? No thank you to this stupid service.”

But if you now understood that he only makes 5% of the scratches and each scratch is followed by a little bump, you would understand that he absolutely a auto-quack and you would run away screaming. And if you had energy you would also complain about him to the auto-painters association.

So the cunning, completely talentless, and irresponsible auto painter will persuade you to buy a service by saying: “All cars will be better (but only statistically so there is no guarantee), and dents are rare (but if it happens, there is nothing I can do about it).

So now you know how to sell stuff; and you also know how to sell chemical medicines. And you know how a pharmaceutical product catalog is written.

You know why you never get the NNTs of the medicines in the catalog, but only the horizontal rapports on mean benefits for the patients; while you systematically will find the NNHs in the catalog.

The auto painter which only makes every 20th scratch and dents every 11th car will tell you now that "all cars I'm working on become better, but between 1% and 10% of the cars will get some dents". You would suffocate him, when you find out how it really is – when you realize how much he has cheated you!

From his sales talk you came to believe that the product was something else, namely that it actually did something good for your car. But everything you bought for your money was invisible paint and maybe a few dents. You have been so badly deceived.

The pharmaceutical catalog is engineered to precisely do this. It is so cleverly done that neither doctors nor patients can see through it. It's pure psychology. The pharmaceutical company gets the pills to look effective and almost harmless. That is the trick. Do you have a product catalog burn it. The information in it is not reliable. It will mislead you. It's a sales brochure not a book of science and objective information. And what it tries to sell you is poisonous. Highly poisonous.

CONCLUSION

Search www.pubmed.gov when you need information about pharmaceutical drugs. Always start to see if there is a Cochrane analysis or another type of meta-analysis or review of the drugs you are recommended for your clinical condition. There is only this way to the most objective information on the chemical products.

All these meta-analyses is still built on RCTs so if you believe in our criticism of the standard RCT method, the Cochrane analysis that in a way just present the combined results from many RCTs will be of little help.

What you must do is to examine whether there is a credible mechanism behind a substance; an antibiotic drug can kill a bacteria if it is sensitive to this particular drug (penicillin against syphilis). If you are missing a substance such as iron, a hormone or a vitamin it is prudent to take this drug when your need has been documented, etc.

Use your common sense and talk to your doctor. If he is a good person and gives you credible explanations of how the substance work, try it and see if it helps. Do not you believe the legend, the label on the glass. If your drug has an NNT of 10, 20 or 50, or figures indicating a 5% or 10% improvement on average, think about what you would do if it was about your car. Or about a hole in the roof of your house. If the hole is 5% smaller after the repair the hole is still almost as big as before, and the rain will still enter. Don't accept that kind of service; it will not help you.

It does not help that we allow our anxiety and other difficult emotions to run the show; such feelings are always found in abundance when we become sick. Common sense is the only way forward, also when it comes to medicine. You might get a friend to support you in taking the choice that is the right for you, especially when those choices are really hardcore. What they almost always are when it comes to disease and death.

Chapter 10

BIOMEDICINE AND HOLISTIC MEDICINE IN CONFLICT

INTRODUCTION

Our Research Clinic for Holistic Medicine was established in 1997, on the shoulders of almost a decades of research in quality of life and strategies for quality of life improvement, and countless of clinical experiments with *quality of life as medicine* (319-321). We were strong believers in CAM – alternative medicine – before 2004. This year we made an extremely thorough and expensive experiment together with the University Hospital in Odense. We tried to treat whiplash patients in a randomised, controlled clinical study using a combination of the very best alternative treatments on the market in Denmark. We invited the best and most acknowledged teachers of the leading CAM schools to join the experiment and we succeeded in getting the very best CAM therapists in Denmark to do the therapy.

We were very excited about this experiment. For the first time we would be able to document that CAM was really working! Unfortunately the results did not agree. Neither the patients' symptoms nor the patients' quality of life were significantly improved (244). Our disappointment was overwhelming. As the honest researchers we are we published our negative results. We knew the results would be quoted by the press and put us in a bad light. And they did. We then fired all the CAM therapists working at the Research Clinic of Holistic Medicine. We changed our treatment strategy and turned to the classical clinical medicine, the Hippocratic holistic medicine, and included the dimension of sexuality that was an important aspect of this medicine.

We also changed the name of the clinic to Research Clinic for Holistic Medicine and Sexology. We simply had to find back to the roots of medicine, to the classical holistic medicine, and the classical principles of healing. We (SV) took at that time the European master degree in CAM (EU-MSc-CAM). We identified from this curriculum and other sources five central principles for holistic healing, which made us understand what the therapists had done wrong in the CAM experiment. Basically we had not taken the patients to existential healing. The whole process was very painful and very enlightening.

With the revival of the classical holistic system of healing, which had a surprisingly strong emphasis on sexuality in line with the philosophy and thinking of psychoanalytic and psychodynamic therapy. And after more than 10 years of research we finally were able to get the medicine to work.

In 2005 and 2006 we were able to document that every second patient we intended to treat for physical, mental, existential, or sexual health issues was cured (60-62,112-116). To our surprise this could be done with only about 20 sessions (one year) of therapy. No doubt we had found back to the roots of medicine. It had been a long, difficult journey, but finally we had found home. The year after we also succeeded in helping half of our patients unable to work or study back to their work or study (117). This was amazing.

As you can imagine our breakthrough, which soon got publicly known as our clinic at that time was very famous in Denmark, also gave us all kinds of problems with the established biomedicine. It was as if it could tolerate a harmless and inefficient CAM but not a highly efficient, sexually oriented, holistic medicine.

Three psychiatrists shared their opinion on our work with the public: It was sexual abuse of the patients! The scandal rolled on the front pages of the boulevard press for days. In the end the police investigated the whole thing, talked to almost all our patients, and concluded after what they called “a very thorough investigation” that “all patients had had a good treatment and some had even been cured” (322).

In 2006 we established the International Campus of Interuniversity College in Copenhagen (225,323), and the first author of this book was appointed the director. At the same time, the National Board of Health removed his medical license temporarily, “as the safety of the holistic treatments needed to be investigated”. To answer the question raised by the national Danish Authorities we made a huge review of more than 1000 scientific papers on CAM, psychotherapy and holistic medicine called “A Review of Side Effects and Adverse Events of Non-Drug Medicine” (122).

We looked for serious side effects and negative events provoked by non-drug medicine. We simple did not find one single documented significant side effect. You cannot harm people by talking to them! And if you only touch them gently and after you have been given permission to do so (consent), this is not harmful either. And if you combine talk and touch therapy, this is not harmful either. So non-drug therapy is harmless. Well, we found that one patient in 64.000 actually got a brief reactive psychosis from the therapy, so this can happen. But such a patient – without a previous mental illness - will heal spontaneously in 2-14 days. This rare side effect is inconvenient but not dangerous at all. On the other hand, we were able to document in a meta-analysis that non-drug therapy actually prevents suicide, and does so efficiently (109).

We would never have given priority to this enormous work which took until 2009 to finish, if the national health authorities had not forced us to do so. Was our findings biased? We found a great number of reviews of all kinds of non-drug therapy that already had documented the lack of side effects for each treatment system, so what we really did was that we made a review of the reviews. Working on this level, bias is harder to introduce. So we believe that any other research group that would do the same work would find the same results as us. So we think not.

Holistic medicine has been acknowledged as harmless ever since Hippocrates, who made “Primum non nocere” – first do no harm – his basis of medical ethics. So every holistic doctor since Hippocrates has been aware not to harm his patients. Hippocrates and his students refused to use pharmaceutical drugs; holistic medicine had no plants or remedies for internal use, exactly for this reason: Primum non nocere (3). Hippocrates was famous for his wisdom.

Table 6 (30). The five central principles of holistic healing in clinical medicine, holistic medicine, clinical holistic medicine and CAM

The principle of salutogenesis: the whole person must be healed (existential healing), not only a part of the person. This is done by recovering the sense of coherence, character and purpose of life of the person.
The similarity principle: only by reminding the patient (or his body, mind or soul) of what made him ill, can the patient be cured. The reason for this is that the earlier wound/trauma(s) live in the subconscious (or body-mind).
The Hering's law of cure (Constantine Hering, 1800-1880): that you will get well in the opposite order of the way you got ill.
The principle of resources: only when you are getting the holding/care and support you did not get when you became ill, can you be healed from the old wound.
The principle of using as little force as possible (primum non nocere or first do no harm), because since Hippocrates (460-377 BCE), "Declare the past, diagnose the present, foretell the future; practice these acts. As to diseases, make a habit of two things - to help, or at least to do no harm." it has been paramount not to harm the patient or running a risk with the patient's life or health.

BIOMEDICINE AND HOLISTIC MEDICINE IN CONFLICT

In spite of strong commercial interests in biomedicine we now observe that holistic, complementary and alternative medicine (CAM) are being used more frequently than biomedicine in the western world. Millions of chronic patients that could not be helped by the biomedical drugs shift these years from believing in drugs to believing in non-drug medicine.

Many physicians have also lost faith in pharmaceutical drugs and start to integrate existential psychotherapy, therapeutic touch, mind-body medicine, clinical holistic medicine, classical sexology and other non-drug holistic medicine techniques into their clinical practice. In response strong commercial forces impact the media and national health authorities to promote the use of biomedical drugs as we saw in the last chapter. But it does not stop there.

Holistic physicians, psychosocial medical researchers, sexologists, CAM-researchers, CAM-therapists and most other categories of non-drug health practitioners are frequently "quack-busted" by their biomedical colleagues following a rigid pattern:

1) First a fabricated accusation is presented to the public and the health authorities via the media,
2) This starts a public investigation often conducted by biomedical doctors, who are strongly biased against holistic medicine and CAM
3) The accusations of malpractice, sexual or violent abuse make some insecure patients re-interpret the treatment and complain about the treatment in the media (they also get fame, money and other privileges in this phase)
4) As this feedback-loop takes off more and more "evidence" gathers against the psychosocial researcher or therapist culminating in a public "witch burning" scandal
5) Even if investigations by the police and the court of law show that the original accusations was unsubstantiated – which is normally the case - the researcher or

therapist will still be found guilty in some level of malpractice by his biomedical collogues based on "moral arguments".

6) In the end the prosecution process generates by itself the evidence against the holistic physician, psychosocial researcher or CAM-therapist that takes him out of business and
7) The national health authorities' participation in the persecution of psychosocial researchers and therapists based on rumors violates the physician and therapist basic human rights and is a serious hindrance to research and development of holistic non-drug medicine.

Many of the leading researchers in holistic medicine have been persecuted for no reason at all except their annoying success with non-drug medicine. The rule is that if a clinical researcher manages to document that he or she can help patients effectively with non-drug medicine this researcher will be in great difficulties shortly after. We know brilliant researchers who even had to flee their country. Wilhelm Reich is one example. He was even thrown into prison for his treatments with body psychotherapy; and he died miserably in that prison only 60 years old. It is not so easy to be pioneer.

How Big Pharma suppresses its opponents

Two industries have economies larger than even small countries: the weapon industry and the biomedical industry. The most powerful way to influence the modern world is by money. Money is God. The sharing of the gigantic turnover from the pharmaceutical industry have been so efficient that it had gained a high popularity. In this process the physician has been the small player; Ross Scholes said it this way: "The highly trained medical professionals is like an accessory to the vast pharmaceutical and health-care industry, as a stewardess is to a jet airliner and the aviations industry" (216,p.37).

It is not completely true that the modern biomedical physician is only serving the pharmaceutical industry; many doctors know that biomedicine like penicillin is highly efficient for syphilis and other life threatening infections but every doctor also seem to agree that drugs have its severe limitations when it comes to curing chronic pain and chronic diseases in general (2).

Recently many physicians has realized that biomedicine is not the only kind of medical science, but when they went to medical school they were only trained to give "the magic bullet" - the pill - and therefore they are not able to understand the process of holistic and existential healing. Therefore they cannot offer the patients psychodynamic psychotherapy, holistic mind-body medicine or any other type of efficient, scientific holistic medicine. They are trapped. To work the way they would like to they need a completely new education in therapy. Which means years without salary. Most physicians that realize that drugs are not the answer to most diseases continues to use the drugs for the rest of the carrier. They are stuck. In Denmark 50% or so of the GPs use CAM in the clinic also, as documented by VIFAB, but the CAM-methods like acupuncture (taken into use after a tree day course in London!) are often only little effective. Fortunately many universities now include courses in holistic medicine which empowers the physician to work with non-drug holistic medicine if he or she prefers that. Most universities in the USA now have courses in mind-body medicine[226]. What a privileged new generation of doctors. But at many universities the battle is still going on. Should we have holistic medicine in the curriculum or not? We cross our fingers that they all in the end will say yes.

Strong commercial interests promote drugs, but a growing number of physicians believe that holistic medicine would help the patient more than the drugs. The reason for this shift in belief is obvious: In countries with nationalized biomedicine, like in Denmark, where all ill people having a chronic disease are treated with drugs at no cost for them the drugs hardly ever cure a patient[2].

Quite on the contrary literally half the nation has been turned into chronic patients: 40-60% of the Danish population is chronically ill now, half with mental and half with somatic illnesses in spite of the free biomedical healthcare (2). For these patients the non-drug therapies are the only alternative. Therefore even physicians now take complementary education in scientific CAM, like the European Master of Science degree (MSc) in complementary, psychosocial and integrative medicine, which has become increasingly popular (225).

ATTACKS ON THE PSYCHOSOCIAL MEDICAL RESEARCHERS AND PRACTITIONERS

In spite of non-drug holistic medicine being helpful and not harmful with sometimes biomedicine being the opposite, biomedicine has managed not only to survive, but also to repress the majority of the psychosocial physicians and researchers on this planet. When you compare the NNT (number needed to treat) and NNH (number needed to harm) for biomedicine and holistic medicine (Chapter 7), remembering that all modern physicians have sworn to rational and evidence-based medicine, this is a riddle.

But when you look to the formation of public consciousness in different societies, you will soon realize that the media is running the show. The media including newspapers, magazines, radio, TV, internet etc. are not only bringing the pharmaceutical industry's massive marketing campaigns paid with literally hundreds of billions of dollar every year; they also constantly bringing hero-stories of doctors saving their patients with brilliant new research and drugs into the media. Big Pharma is very skilled in using journalists for hidden marketing.

But the activities are not only about securing that the positive message gets out. As important is the negative message about its competitors. And the industry obviously takes holistic medicine as a real threat and treats it accordingly.

The media bring one story after the other on "CAM-quacks" harming, violating and abusing their patients, which make the population insecure about this kind of medicine, so that biomedicine and the pharmaceutical industry will stay in power and hold its position on the market. And sell more drugs next year.

Most interestingly it seems that the pharmaceutical industry has found an ingenious solution to the threat from complementary and holistic medicine: *Directing whom the public health care system will investigate*. The process can be small and invisible for the public with some accusations of violations, medical errors, and harm done to a patient, making it justified that the health authorities look into the practice of the holistic doctor, CAM-researcher or sexologist, finding all the things that can be criticized, especially all the things that deviate from the "rational" *biomedical standard treatment.*

The publicly employed medical experts that evaluate a controversial holistic medicine research or treatment are normally biomedical doctors, often biomedical psychiatrists with a collective, close link to the pharmaceutical industry, and no understanding of or sympathy for CAM or holistic medicine. The physician practicing non-drug medicine will therefore end up being blamed in public for not treating correctly according to standard. Even if the holistic medicine treatment is done as research, this fact that it is research, which would fully explain the found divergence from standard treatment, will often be denied.

The political system, which is under severe pressure from the biomedical pharmaceutical lobby, often accepts "preponderance of evidence" against the non-drug therapist and finds him guilty. In the recent period, when these cases have been brought in front of the court system (not the medical system) with demands of "clear and convincing evidence", then the therapist is almost always found not-guilty (324). But then the harm is already done.

WITCH HUNTING IN THE MEDIA

Often the opponents of holistic medicine are using the media to obtain the intended public investigation. Most often biomedical physicians, again often psychiatrists, go to the media with severe accusations of malpractice, sexual and violent abuse, horrible errors and serious harm done by the non-drug therapist.

The media often buy into the stories, as sex, violence and news connected to medicine attracts enormous attention and sell newspapers more than anything else. Afterwards the public health authorities are politically motivated to engage and demonstrate strength and efficiency by attacking the CAM-therapist, revoking license etc. Often "leaks" to the media from the investigating biomedical doctors who often are strongly biased against holistic medicine will bring a continuous flow of hot stories about the "bad" doctor/therapist.

As soon as a non-drug therapist is brought in this position, his patients lose faith and confidence, and often they start re-interpreting what actually happened in the clinic and can even complain over the treatment, often directly motivated by the media hunting the good story, in spite of feeling helped and completely satisfied with the treatment only yesterday.

A strong wish to distance them and to get rid of an embarrassing association with the quack and "CAM-witch" it often what makes them terminate their treatment and change their opinion of the non-drug therapist. This is a normal psychological mechanism; we know from the New Testament that even the disciples of Jesus repudiated him, when he was caught by the Romans to be crucified. We should expect less stamina from our vulnerable patients.

Even in the unlikely case that the CAM-therapist or holistic doctor is a true saint, a strong negative campaign in the media will still make him look like a criminal. So the strongly negative, evil-intended exposure of the non-drug therapist, most often with fabricated evidences and untrue accusations, will destroy the therapist's name and clinical practice. The national health authorities could save a good doctor by investigating the case that is brought to attention in the media, and tell everybody what they found out; but this is not how it works.

It seems the reality around a government is too politically and financially motivated to be guided primarily by truth and honesty. Instead of investigating the actual case, the public organs normally start to investigate the non-drug therapist himself. They normally go through all his case-records, many hundred of them, to see if he has done some errors in the past. Often this investigation goes back for many years. And the criteria for an error is seldom that a patient were harmed, or not helped; even if every single patient is helped and perfectly satisfied, the holistic physician will be blamed that he is not treating according to normal "biomedical standard".

The patients who start complaining will win their cases just because of this, in spite of knowing what treatment they originally accepted, and in spite of this treatment actually helping them. Most sadly, as soon as the therapist is seen as a non-healing and a destructive, harmful therapist, much of the therapeutic gain is actively destroyed by the patients, to disengage and distance him or herself from the therapist. So many hours and years of good therapeutic work with the patients can be wasted in a single evil campaign. Non-drug intervention is always using the placebo effects, and the "nocebo effect" is as strong, just reversed. So the patients can easily destroy their therapeutic gains.

The double fork-attack by the media and the public health authorities are mutually reinforcing each other, making life a true hell for the non-drug therapist, who can literally lose everything in a few days or weeks. Non-drug therapists who experience this are often forced to flee their own country, and in practice almost all basic human rights are seriously violated (70 see appendix).

It is worth to underline that it is the national health authorities that have the faith of the citizens, as it is normally expected that these national organs are there for the sake of the citizens. Everybody knows of course that the boulevard press or media are living from lies about sex, violence and all evil. So the responsibility for the massive violation of the human rights of the CAM-therapists is really with the national health agencies.

Witch burning/hunting of the holistic doctor or CAM-therapists is a social phenomenon fueled by a combination of several strong interests in society: The people want entertainment, and this must be about sex, violence, abuse, failure etc. The "evil doctor" abusing his patients is one of the archetypical stories that never stops entertaining. The media makes lots of money on twisting reality and adding sex and violence to the stories and the best stories are about people pretending to do good, but instead being sexually violent and abusive. Our unconscious shadow likes such stories.

Holistic medicine, sexology, and the efficient types of CAM-therapy are by nature strongly provocative to the patients' emotions and feelings; all mind-body medicine has in general a body-and sex positive attitude. Holistic medicine has lots of enemies, like the competitive pharmaceutical companies, the biomedical physicians, conservative, materialistic people in high-power positions in society etc.

Witch burning of holistic physicians, researchers and CAM-therapists often involve politicians taking a free ride to exploit the situation and gain political position and power. This often leads to strong activation of public health organizations to investigate and even arrest the therapist and a strong motivation to "safe the patients" by proving his guilt. Often this process creates its own evidence against the holistic therapists, very much like the famous processes against the witches did five hundred years ago.

In the process of being torched as a "witch" the psychosocial therapist or researcher often looses all human rights, all material and intellectual properties, and in the end as mentioned even his country.

He often ends up like a refugee, who not even in the neighboring countries can live and practice his non-drug therapy or research. Even if the therapist in the end of the process wins in the court of law (as is often the case) and all accusations turn out to be false, he will often have lost everything, because of his bad public standing.

It is most problematic that which-burning seems to be systematically used as a weapon against the psychosocial non-drug therapists and researchers in processes started all over the world by powerful organizations like the *Quackwatch* which seemingly being used by the pharmaceutical industry to silence and pacify (the industry call it "neutralize" and "discredit" (157)) its enemies (217). It is therefore important that every person professionally involved in health and justice understands the mechanism of witch-burning to avoid participating in it.

WHAT SHOULD BE DONE?

To prevent the national health authorities violating the basic human rights of the CAM-therapist, holistic doctors, and researchers in holistic medicine that destroys good therapists and research that the country desperately needs and hinder the development of medicine into a more efficient, more holistic, and less harmful medicine, it is absolutely necessary that:

The national authority only investigate the actual case or complaint, and only find such a complain substantiated by facts when there is "clear and convincing evidence", and not only "preponderance of evidence". If the error is found to be substantiated by a competent organ, presumably the court of law, and only if it is found to be harmful to patients, and likely to be representative of more similar errors done by the therapist, only then there is a reason to investigate the general practice of the non-drug therapist or researcher.

All investigations should be done in absolute confidentiality regarding the public and the media, and in complete openness regarding the holistic doctor or CAM-therapist, who must be heard before any decision regarding the (mal)treatment is made.

Educated experts in CAM and holistic medicine, not biomedical experts and psychiatrists likely to be biased against non-drug medicine, must do the investigation. In Europe for example we have the Master of Science in complementary, psychosocial and integrative medicine at the Interuniversity College in Graz based on a dedicated and long non-drug practice. There are hundreds of competent people with this master that can be asked for assistance.

Sexual abuse can in therapy happen in spite of consent as it per definition is abuse when a physician/therapist has sex with a patient (129). It is important to notice that sex means coitus, cunnilingus or fellatio, or the patient for any reason touching the therapist's naked genitals. If these kinds of sexual behavior are not present, the patient has not been sexually abused per definition. The reason for such a strict definition is the need for the physician to be able to talk freely about sexuality and to use all available, gynecological procedures and all sexological tools, including bodywork like the sexological examination to help his patient.

The ethical code can also be violated in spite of no harm done. We strongly recommend the ethical code of the International Society for Holistic Health (129).

CONCLUSIONS

Holistic medicine is the original medicine, a psychosocial medicine that has been used for thousands of years and is highly effective. Today industrial medicine has almost completely displaced it to an almost forgotten position. The physicians have for a generation or so not been trained in psychosocial medicine but the last two or three decades non-drug medicine has again been highly popular with the patients. Unfortunately the physicians cannot provide it, but most universities in USA have now included courses in mind-body medicine into the curriculum, and medical schools in Europe are following, so the next generation of physicians will be able to provide this classical and harmless medicine again.

The development has been seen as a threat by the pharmaceutical industry and the biomedical physicians it collaborate with. It has been suggested that the pharmaceutical industry has developed into a sort of mafia (220), but we don't think it is a mafia in that Russian sense. It is more like a materialist belief in chemistry and DNA that for many years has been associated with power and money, which attracts a special segment of the physicians, who then get very rich and powerful. The problem is that chemical medicine is less good for the patients' health than it is for the physician's prestige, wealth and academic position. Biomedical drugs have systematically failed to cure the patients and one in two of the Danes are chronically ill (2). It is time to realize that health cannot be bought for money. It takes human contact, lowing care, deep talks and exploration within, to heal a wounded body or soul.

As non-drug therapy is not dangerous or harmful the biomedical physicians should stop creating all sorts of wild stories and rumors about "the danger of CAM" and the national health agencies should also stop persecuting the providers and researchers of holistic medicine.

The wise national health agency will understand that talk touch therapy is often effective and always harmless and in this understanding they will abstain from blaming the therapists and researchers, even when biomedical colleagues or organizations closely related to the pharmaceutical industry make accusations. In spite of the small likelihood of a therapist causing harm there might be occasions where it is appropriate to investigate but this investigation most be done discretely, as the knowledge of a clinic or therapist being investigated is very embarrassing and make many patients react negatively.

In the case of a holistic physician, sexologist or CAM-therapist being accused by biomedical colleagues – or by patients for that sake - he or she is innocent until proven guilty. The media can often destroy a CAM-therapist's or clinical researcher's whole clinical practice together with the therapeutic gains of his patients with stories just based on rumors and suspicions. There should be laws against that but such are difficult to have in a country with free speech.

The national authorities that have the trust of the people should under no circumstances engage in such evil-intended campaigns as we have seen it happen in Denmark. The national health agencies should do their very best to be informed about CAM and holistic medicine, and if there is a complaint they should not share any suspicion with the public. They should announce faults and harm, when they are certain to have happened, but not before.

To secure that the citizens get the best medicine possible, and that all controversies are given a fair process in the public system it is extremely important that governments and their organizations and employees keep clear of every connection to the pharmaceutical industry, financially and otherwise. Public hospitals and universities should not receive findings from the pharmaceutical industry; is it necessary for the industry to pay this money should be collected as taxes, to remove the power from the industry.

Only when experts in holistic medicine are evaluating other holistic therapists and researchers can the evaluation be fair and unbiased. This does not mean that acupuncturists must evaluate acupuncturists, but the evaluating person must be a trained holistic physician, sexologist or CAM-therapist. He or she must be scientifically trained in the healing principles of holistic medicine.

Chapter 11

How do we develop medicine from being poisonous drugs into being an efficient and safe medicine?

The world is in a chaotic state, and money rules. Many people have been mislead and information has been withheld. The RCT method has not only been manipulated in hundred small ways to introduce huge biases some of which can be removed in Cochrane metaanalyses (the biases related to the statistical analysis of the data, not the biases related to the production of the raw data). The RCT method has been set up so helpful that any poisonous drug will come out as efficient and almost harmless medicine. Of course it is still an art to find drugs that are not so harmful that they kill the patient, so lots of test animals are sacrificed in this process. But basically this is a mess.

Huge amount of money is harvested on drugs that are really doubtful, like the Swine Flu vaccine given for a mild type of influenza. Maybe we even need these infections for our immune system to prepare for the next more fatal influenza type?

And huge amounts of money come from the sales of anti-depressive and anti-psychotic drugs, which according the Cochrane analyses we have presented is not improving mental health (the patients' mental state).

And huge amounts of money come from anti-cancer chemotherapy, in spite of the fact that Abel found it harmful for most types of cancers.

And money flows continuously from other products like penicillin given to children with acute otitis, NSAID painkillers for arthritis etc which are not very helpful either, as we have seen.

The pharmaceutical companies market their product aggressively and often illegal as we have seen, and even the national drug directories which are based on national medicine agencies guiding all physicians and patients contain data from the industry only, and not the more valid data from the Cochrane metaanalyses and other independent researchers.

In the same time we have CAM often not working, and classical holistic medicine and sexology that are almost forgotten and also quite border transgressing for patients and people who has got accustomed to the nice, clean, polite way of the biomedical doctors. In a way it is so much nicer to give patients pills than to confront them with their existential problems they are trying to escape by all means. You can be distant and polite when you give pills; but when you give love you need closeness and intimacy. And this is what we fear more than anything.

Because this takes us to our feelings. And we don't like that because this is where we as modern people have our real problems. Holistic medicine is about feeling, about healing wounded feelings. It is about taking the patients back to their childhood to reshape their personality. It is bloody. It is hard. It is painful. It is shameful. It is all that we neurotically try to avoid.

So it is really easy for people who not think too much to like biomedicine, to prefer a treatment with drugs, instead of a treatment based on introspection and existential exploration. We understand that. Believe us, we do.

But the consequences of the state of things are devastating. According to the statistics[182] about 50% of the Danish population takes drugs regularly. When we compare to the Cochrane metaanalyses we estimate that about half of these drugs are much less effective and much more harmful than listed in the Danish national drug directory. We estimate from this comparative analysis that about 25% of the drugs are only harmful; they have no specific beneficial qualities at all. But this is if we accept the RCT method at scientifically sound and valid. This means that about 1/8 of the whole population or about 700.000 people every day take a drug that is only harmful and not beneficial for them. Many of these patients, presumably more than 200.000 a year, will get adverse effects, and undoubtedly many of these patients will also die or lose some important abilities for life. So many people are harmed that this is a treat to our collective thriving and survival. It is really a serious threat to our society. On a global scale this is a treat to our world.

But then, if we take it to the next level, and reject the RCT procedure in this book, as we have done, things get really dark. Now, what is happening in the factories of the pharmaceutical industry is no longer rational and fine science. It is only looking like medical science. In reality it is just applied chemistry where poisonous drugs are made to look like beneficial almost harmless medicine, and sold to the trustful, vulnerable sick patients though the person they trust the most: Their doctor. This becomes unbearable, does it not?

And what is happening is that almost all the money that is made is returned to market the drugs in direct and indirect ways. Only a few percent is collected as profit. But a few percent of an incredible number of billions of dollars is still OK. Especially as the turnover groves 10-20% a year, and has done that for decades, and seem to continue, until Big Pharma owe the whole world. Which will happen pretty soon if we don't wake up. And at that point in time no democratic processes can stop it anymore. Today this will already be a hard battle that even might take whole governments down. But in 10 or 20 years this battle can no longer be won. So we need to take it now.

So the world is burning. And this is smartly done. Almost no people see the danger. Very few people realize what is happening. Everybody wants to believe in our society, our government, our industry that gives us all the nice jobs, and in medical science which the industry promises soon will cure cancer and everything bad. It is just a question of few years now. As it has been for 50 years now.

We, the independent medical scientists, know how things are - from our perspective. And maybe we are nuts, crazy, just fruitcakes, as the opponents of non-drug medicine often say we are. The biomedical psychiatrists that hate CAM and holistic medicine and classical sexology and everything that comes close to feelings and bodily touch.

But maybe we are the sane people in a crazy world, the whistleblowers you need to pay attention to, because we are in the burning room in the basement of the building, and you are not. We have seen the flames, but you have hardly noticed the smoke yet. They time you do it might very well be too late. So maybe you need to listen to our whistle which we today blow as hard as we can.

WHAT WE WANT TO TELL YOU

We do not want to go to the extreme as to abandon pharmaceutical drugs completely. We strongly believe that many of them are helpful, at least for a short period of time, or to cure an acute disease like Syphilis, Boreliosis, and Meningitis. So our errand is not to close the pharmaceutical industry but to ensure for the world that we only use drugs that really are helpful. And only use them when it is helpful. And only for so long as it is helpful.

In our own Research Clinic for Holistic Medicine and Sexology, we have only prescribed drugs to 2% of our more than 500 patients. The rest of the patients have been treated with non-drug medicine. In a normal biomedical clinic about 90% of the patients get pharmaceutical drugs. We found that half of our patients got cured, independent of the diagnosis, as we have seen. So we believe that the use of drugs could be reduced with about 98% in general practice, and that this would be extremely helpful for the patients. We were grateful that we had the drugs for the about 2% of the patients that needed them – penicillin, morphine, antihistamine, antifungal drugs etc. It was good for them. In the end it was not the drugs that cured them; when they got in better balance their immune system got better so they were able to win the battle against the microorganism themselves; and their soul as well as their muscles relaxed so their chronic pain disappeared. Holistic medicine cured them. But the drugs were very helpful in the acute phase of the illness. So we want the drugs to be on the market. All the drugs that can help. We only need to be absolutely certain that the drugs are helpful to the patients, as we know for sure that they are *poisonous*.

We believe that most readers by now realize that we cannot continue to let the pharmaceutical industry test their own pharmaceutical products. This is crazy. The industry is to biased, to dishonest, too involved in making money, to do this in a way that can be trusted. This is why the metaanalysis systematically documents less positive effect and more harm than the pharmaceutical industry, as we have seen. And then we have the problem of the invalid RCT-test. Which is even a harder problem. For the pharmaceutical industry is not likely to accept this test as invalid. If they do they are forced to accept that their drugs are tested in comparison with holistic non-drug medicine. Because to harvest NNTs and NNHs in such trials is the only way to test the drugs fairly; and it is highly likely that only a few percent of the drugs will survive such a comparative test. These are the drugs that we actually needs.

We need independent organs to test the pharmaceutical drugs. This is not a simple thing, for who can be independent when the pharmaceutical industry has grown to this tremendous size? When it has its people and its money everywhere?

In Denmark we have the National Medicines Agency (Lægemiddelstyrelsen) under the National Board of Health (Sundhedsstyrelsen). But these organs are, as we have seen, NOT providing the physicians or the patients with the information about the positive effect (the Number Needed to Treat, or NNT) and adverse effects and events (the Number Needed to Harm, or NNH) for the different outcomes for each drug tested.

On the contrary it seems that these official organs cooperate perfectly with the pharmaceutical companies in keeping these numbers secret. The reason for this secrecy is obvious. Who would take a normal drug if it only helps 5% of the patients (NNT=20) and at the same time harms 33% or more of the patients (NNH_{total}=1-3)?

And if people understood that they are not cured by these drugs but that they most likely will become chronic patients for life, if they rely on the drugs to cure them, would they then take them - or would they seek some alternative, holistic treatment with higher likelihood to cure? You see? This is quite logical. The information needs to be kept secret for the biomedical system – the whole medico-industrial complex - to continue its activities and growths.

The whole drug business can only work when the true information is kept secret for the health politicians, the doctors and the patients, and the massively manipulating marketing machinery at the same time makes every single patient and citizen believe that *everybody* is helped by the drugs (!) and almost nobody is harmed by the pharmaceutical drugs.

If you analyze any biomedical commercial you will find that this basically is the message repeated again and again and again by every single commercial from the pharmaceutical industry. 1500 times a year. Again and again and again. Until people believe it.

Which people eventually will as nobody contradicts it or criticizes it; not even the employees at the National Medicines Agency and National Health Agency which are the organs installed by the government to protect the people from the dark side of the commercial medicines' interests. This is truly horrible. This is worst case scenario. Big Pharma has almost won the whole world. Thousands of medical doctors that wants a more objective and fair evaluation of the drugs' effects engage in the national Cochrane Centers and other independent research organizations, like The Quality of Life Research Center in Copenhagen, Denmark, or the National Institute of Child Health and Human Development in Israel.

But what can a few thousand honest physicians do against Big Pharma with its immensely huge complex of gifts, sponsorships, advertisements, lobbyism, scientific manipulations, withhold of vital information from the public, methodological fraud, political deceptions and bold lies about the effects and harms of the drugs we are up against here? Not much. We need you to engage also. We need politicians to join. We need more than anything decent and honest, brave (very brave) journalists to participate in the battle and *start to inform people about the state of things*. We need consciousness about this. We need light. Sharp analysis. Clever journalism. Brave hearted politicians that cannot and will not accept that 10% of the total population or more is harmed by the products of the pharmaceutical industry every year.

The experiences from Denmark have taught us clearly that the National Health Agency and the National Medicine Agency have not had the political power to withstand the pressure from the pharmaceutical industry. 20 years ago critical researchers developed a fine understanding in bias of randomised clinical trials (67).

It was clear from this research that there was more than hundred different ways a clinical drug test could be manipulated to show a better result than it should. The national health agencies made rules to cope with that, and scientific ethical committees we asked to approve the industrial research protocols to avoid fraud and manipulations. But it did not take long before all the seats in these organs were occupied with biomedical doctors and academic professors from institutions close to or even co-funded by the pharmaceutical industry.

As we have seen the pharmaceutical industry has continued to improve and refine the RCT, until it was turned into the perfect tool for getting drugs approved it is today. Even drugs that have no specific pharmacological beneficial effect – drugs that only are poisons – can now be approved as effective and rational medicine with this method, as we have seen many examples of in this book.

All this time the national organs which should have controlled the pharmaceutical industry have been fast asleep. And so Big Pharma got its way.

The market has been drowned in pharmaceutical products that independent research centers have found to be only harmful. I am sure that these researchers have informed these organs personally – as we have. In spite of this, these harmful drugs stay on the market.

The results of the Cochrane Metaanalysis are completely ignored; large independent studies of the effect of Chemotherapy – and many other drugs for that sake – that document that these drugs kill patients and destroy their quality of life are simply ignored! Obviously this is happening because of politics and money. What is this for a world! How brutal, dirty, selfish a world, how predatory an industry.

The Cochrane Metaanalyses are also often biased – in favour of the drugs. Often they contain data, as we have seen, which justifies the conclusion that the drugs should be withdrawn from the market immediately. But the abstract do almost never say that, in spite of this information about the drugs being harmful and not beneficial in the papers. The political pressure on the Cochrane centers is immense. We have heard about the English Cochrane researcher Tom Jefferson receiving murder threats from the Influenza vaccine industry, but this is only one story out of a hundred that could be told of this kind. A Swedish TV-documentary team that exposed a pharmaceutical company had to live under cover for years (325). This is not the place to list all the bad things that has happens to the independent researchers and journalists focusing on the pharmaceutical industry; interested readers can get more info in our paper addressing this specific problem (70). Just know that this is hardball.

We obviously need a completely new organ to test the therapeutic value of medicine, with employees that in no way are connected with the pharmaceutical industry or biomedicine, to test the drugs. If such a test organ was given the power and resources to really control the drugs independently, it could in a few years remove the inefficient and harmful drugs from the market, including the bad drugs we have mentioned in this book: the anti-depressive medicine (132), the antipsychotic medicine (133), the chemotherapy for most types of cancers (82), the wrongly tested influenza vaccines (68,69), the inefficient painkillers (67), and the ineffective penicillin cures for many of the child infection like acute otitis (63).

We have only scratched the surface in our book. We have only mentioned about 10 of almost 10.000 Cochrane meta-analyses. Hundreds of drugs has been analyzed for dozens of clinical conditions, and all this information needs to be integrated in biomedicine medicine.

But then there are a thousand drugs more which all are tested with the flawed RCT procedure. Most of them are likely to go. What would happen if they were tested and found useless as medicine? Imagine the pharmaceutical industry breaking down. Hundreds of thousands of people would lose their jobs. Stockholders and companies all over the world would go bankrupt. Doctors in thousands would be without the drugs they prescribe every single day, and will go out of business. And all the patients would suddenly stand with the responsibility for their own life, which they never have learned to handle. The result is even more chaotic than the present condition. Disaster, depression, crisis will follow. This is worse than recession. No politician in the world would want that to happen. So we might have a problem engaging the politicians in this. See?

Therefore it is time to think about the true values of life. Is it really good for us that our economy is hot, that everybody is busy, that we produce so many things and have so expensive cars and travel so many airplanes and life in so much material luxury, when we pay with our quality of life and our health?

What is most important: Love or money? What is more precious: Life or things? What do you want: Tremendous material wealth and a planet that is not inhabitable by your children's children? Or a sustainable world where everybody is consuming with awareness of the needs of nature and the need of ecological balance of the world? Please wake up. Stop the madness. Get some common sense into the world. We need it urgently. We need it now.

And what about all the madmen – the 6% or so of the population now conveniently drugged down to passivity with anti-psychotic drugs (182)? All the repressed anger and hatred that will explode in our heads the moment the chemical thigh jackets are removed? Should we build a thousand more prisons for these people? And what about all the desperate depressed people and cancer patients who now at least live in the hope of betterment, how little justified this hope might be; should we just let them fall down in the darkness of hopelessness and despair?

It is quite obvious that we cannot take biomedicine away without substituting the drugs with something else. Fortunately we have a highly developed holistic medicine ready to take over. We have all the knowledge from the old Hippocratic and pre-modern traditions of healing and medicine; we have many different cultures' medicine system intact.

To make it simple we could easily in just a few years train a million physicians and medical students in using the classical methods of Hippocrates holistic medicine. Our group has during the last ten years written a number of textbooks that could be used, and many more could be written. The knowledge is there. Just go to www.pubmed.gov and make a search for "holistic medicine" and see what can be cured this way. It's amazing. This jewel of medical knowledge is not used today, this golden treasury of knowledge on healing and personal development. But it could be. It should be. It is just a question of political will.

We find it highly problematic that the best and most recognized scientific journals of medicine – like The Lancet, JAMA, New England Journal of Medicine, BMJ - are not objective in spite of their intentions to be so but often also biased towards biomedicine and drugs. We hope that it is only a question of time before these mastodons wake up and realize their duty to free the people of the world from the burden of poisoning they also have a shared responsibility of causing as they have accepted the many drug-papers based on the flawed RCT method. When they understand what they have been doing, these intelligent editors, they cannot continue their conservative practice that favors the drugs.

Paradoxically we find nothing wrong with science itself; the sciences of chemistry, biochemistry, cell biology, physiology etc are all valid and necessary for medicine. All the subjects taught at med school are all right in themselves. These subjects are actually very important to understand biology, to get a deep, scientific understanding of how the body is build and functions.

The problem is not what is taught in med school. The problem is what is NOT taught. We did not have one single lecture of existential healing and salutogenesis during our whole medical education.

Not one single hour were we told about what the physicians did before the drugs became the medicine of the world. If we had know that such a thing as existential healing (salutogenesis) actually existed, that it was not just a joke about crazy CAM people believing in strange zones under the feet and mysterious energy fields not likely to exist at all etc. we would have started healing our patients right away.

Not telling us that patients could be healed was the reason we believed in drugs to being with. This was the crime: Not sharing the treasure of medicine with us as students. And this is what has to be changed in the future. We are sure that the physicians would like to heal their patients. Absolutely sure. And we are absolutely certain that the patients will prefer a cure addressing the cause of the disease for a mere blocking of the symptoms any time. At least if they are correctly informed about the possibilities and the prospects for the patients with the alternative treatments, biomedicine and holistic medicine.

Today many health politicians know that there is so much more health and healing for a dollar in holistic medicine than in pharmaceutical drugs. The info we gave you in chapter 7 is well known to the experts. But being a politician is about what is practically possible, not about utopia.

The moment people wake up and realize what is going on regarding biomedicine the voters will go for a change. The voters will go for a safe and efficient medicine without drugs. We believe it is time for the politicians to enter the fight for a better medicine now. We, the independent researchers, are mobilizing all over the world now. We need politicians to join the battle. We cannot do it alone; we do not as researchers have the strength and the power to win over the pharmaceutical industry's tricks and manipulations. Every day some us are we are defunded, discredited, forced to flee our country and give up our jobs. We need the cavalierly. Come now, please.

If you are dean of a medical faculty, or employed by a university to teach medicine, you can start helping by informing your students and colleagues about the principles and results of holistic medicine and salutogenesis (existential healing). You can even suggest to the dean that holistic medicine becomes a part of the medical curriculum again. Medicine is primarily about humans helping each other, and not about chemistry, however fascinating one can find the natural sciences.

If you are a journalist you have a most important job: Be critical to all the stories brought to you by the people close to the pharmaceutical industry and the biomedical physicians and experts that work with the industry. Whenever you hear a story about a "Quack" that harms his patients by talking with them and touching them therapeutically, please check the story twice or even trice.

As holistic medicine has no known adverse effects (122), as talk and soft touch are completely harmless and non-invasive, don't believe the biomedical psychiatrists and doctors who claim that "this patient went crazy", and "that patient killed herself" because of this treatment. These are the lies so often presented by the people of Big Pharma. Lies that only are produced to harm, repress and destroy CAM and holistic medicine. Don't help them do that. We need good, efficient, sustainable medicine. Not poisonous drugs, more poisonous drugs and yet more poisons.

Please research every story thoroughly and always, always, always follow the money to see who pays. Because the financial interests run the show. Don't serve the dark side. Don't join the dark side. Help making a better world. Don't be servant of money and power. Think. Act differently. Make a difference. Do good. All good hands are needed. We have a huge job to do. Please join us. We are working as hard as we can. But we cannot do it alone.

Chapter 12

CONCLUSION: THE PHARMACEUTICAL INDUSTRY SELLS POISONS AS MEDICINE AND KNOWS THAT THE DOCUMENTATION SHOULD BE BETTER

From our scientific and philosophical position there are several levels of the pharmaceutical industry's deception of the world and its politicians, physicians and patients.

On level of deception is that the pharmaceutical industry is making rocket science. Molecular research is not that complicated. Research in feelings, emotions, consciousness, brain function etc is much more complex and difficult; much more demanding intellectually. Permutating molecules and testing them on animals are not that difficult. It might look impressive with a new molecule in medicine but what it can do for you is rather limited.

Let's take an example. We were all impressed when we first heard about Viagra, because erective dysfunction is tormenting a lot of men and if a pill could solve that problem this would be a remarkable help to these men. But when we later saw the metaanalysis of the clinical trial reports (229) we realized that the company had not really delivered according to the promises (238) mentioned above (Chapter 4). One in three men was able to have intercourse about every second time they tried with Viagra... This is better than nothing, and sure it is, seen from the man's perspective. Much seems to indicate this does not lead to satisfying sex for the woman, who is more sensitive to the emotional problems in the relationship causing the erective dysfunction (240). The sad thing is that we have excellent sexological treatments for male erective dysfunction that in most cases can be permanently cured (NNT=1 (240), NNH=64.000 (122)); in the same time the therapy solves the causal layer of emotional problems that gives both the erective dysfunction, AND the lack of sexual excitement and desire AND the females problems with feelings of loneliness and lack of desire, lubrication, sexual excitement, and orgasmic problems.

So what Viagra does is that is pretends to solve a problem that it does not really solve; it only blocks a part of the symptom; it is correct that one in three men more often can penetrate his women technically, when on the drug but when it comes to sexual happiness and quality of life the drug might even be contraproductive (238). And then we should not forget that there are both physical side effects (NNH=3, NNH_{total}=1-2 (estimated from (229)) and also what could be called philosophical side effects in that the man's focus shifted gets away from the emotional problems to the physical and mechanical level. We find it correct to say that the man in a way get duller and faster asleep existentially when using Viagra, as argued in our paper on Viagra (238).

So this is very much the situation. Life is not so much about the mechanical and chemical level as it is about consciousness, relationships, feelings, love, intimacy, sexual excitement and desire etc. The drugs have physical side effects but the mental and philosophical side effects are even bigger: People who use drugs start to think about the body as a mechanical machine, which it most definitely is not, because it is a biological organism where *biological information* is materialized into form - organs like skin, brain, heart, muscles, and bones. Diseases are caused by disturbances in this biological information system, which then materialize a disturbance in the mind or body. You can easily understand what is going on inside yourself if you understand and trust your feelings. Therefore, everything that takes your focus away from your feelings, existential core, and sense of coherence and direction in life is harming you.

So the chemical level of the medical research is most of the time not really helpful, and much less helpful than we are made to believe. Viagra is one of the most successful of the new drugs, and even this drug seems to have a hard time in competition with the classical holistic sexological methods. Why aren't we happy with the old ways that have helped so many men and women through the ages? Why would we abandon sexology and replace it with drugs? Well, because we are mislead. The information we get points in the chemical direction. Your physician will prescribe you Viagra instead of refereeing to a sexologist because he is mislead and now think that Viagra is a better solution for you as patient. And you might not even have heard about the non-drug treatment for the sexual dysfunctions, as you are not an expert. But you have heard about Viagra. You have heard a lot. For the drug company and its collaborators have planted this story 1000 times in the media already. It is a good story. It sounds so logic: Oh, so I need this molecule to get a hard on. It is so stupid, because sex is a psychosocial and emotional thing, not a mechanical thing. When all the consciousness-stuff is working, the body is ALWAYS fine.

DECEPTION ON THE LEVELS OF BIAS

It has been known for a long time that the pharmaceutical industry is generally not objective when they document the positive and negative effects of its products, the pharmaceutical drugs. All too often severe biases have been found, on all levels of the test used for documenting the drugs: the randomised clinical trial (RCT). There are two major classes of biases, biases related to the phases happening before data analysis, and biases related to the phases after data analysis. When the raw data is analyzed again in metaanalyses using strict protocols most of the second class of bias can be eliminated. When this is done it is often found that the documented positive effects are gone and the adverse effects are increasing dramatically. We have seen this pattern with the anti-cancer chemotherapy and antipsychotic drugs. In the metaanalysis both these classes of drugs were shown not to benefit the patients' health and survival but to harm the patients significantly. Quality of life was destroyed and survival time was shortened. We concluded based on this that the drugs were not useful as medicine. Obviously the positive results found by the pharmaceutical industry was based on bias. But many drugs does still have an effect in the Cochrane metaanalyses after removing (most of) the statistical bias. It is difficult to remove the pre-statistical bias; most likely this will take a completely new study.

DECEPTION ON THE LEVEL OF METHOD

But them there are problems from the RCT itself. If we look at a Cochrane metaanalysis where active placebo is used instead of the normal "passive placebo" we can see that the anti-depressive effect of the anti-depressive drugs is removed. Obviously the whole effect was a product of active placebo destroying the blindness of the study. This means that in RCTs with biologically active drugs the blinding is destroyed as the patients can feel the active drugs, and therefore believe more in being helped than the patients that only got the passive placebo pill (often a piece of sugar or chalk). Based on this we find the whole RCT-procedure to be fake.

When we look carefully after there are three more reasons not to believe in the RCT procedure. All four errors sums up to the fatal error that the RCT test seems to get any poisonous drug turned into a seemingly efficient and harmless chemical medicine.

This means that not only anti-depressive drugs but all drugs that have been tested with the RCT procedure must be suspected to only be poisonous drugs with no specific positive pharmacological effect. The whole project of biomedicine seems to be an illusion. Drugs don't work; they only manipulate our consciousness to believe that they work, and then our consciousness, which in reality controls our health (17), make the drug work. The placebo effect is what is active in medicine. This is in accordance with the understanding of Hippocrates and his students (3). We have also found that consciousness is the primary cause of health and disease, quality of life, ability and many more dimensions of life (17). But this is fundamentally in conflict with the chemical religion of biomedicine (called *monistic materialism* in philosophy).

In our paper in the RCT method (1) and in the first five chapters of this book we have documented that the pharmaceutical industry's standard method for testing the pharmaceutical drugs, the randomised clinical trial (RCT), is so seriously flawed that it cannot be accepted as a scientifically valid method.

The many different forms of bias can easily manipulate the result of the test so radically that it becomes completely misleading, but the inner structure of the RCT-test is much worse: It tends to document systematically that poisons are effective and harmless medicine.

DECEPTION ON THE LEVEL OF INFORMATION – PROMOTING AND REPRESSING INFO

The drugs are marketed aggressively by the pharmaceutical industry, and its allies, the biomedical physicians, as we have seen. Especially the psychiatrists are totally dependent of the psycho-pharmacological drugs as the non-drug medical methods have been completely forgotten in psychiatry. This might explain why the psychiatrists are far the worse to attack the holistic physicians, holistic medical researchers, and CAM therapists.

It is not known in much detail how the destruction and repression of the "enemies" of Big Pharma is carried out, but in connection to the Vioxx scandal the investigators, according to The Australian in April 2009, found "hit lists" listing researchers that should be "neutralized" and "discredited" (157). An internal email from the pharmaceutical company read loud in court said: "We may need to seek them out and destroy them where they live." (157)

The researchers listed on the company's "hit-list" did research in the adverse effects of the drug Vioxx that gave some of the patients acute myocardiac infarction and stroke. Critiques believe that the pharmaceutical company tried to repress this research to keep Vioxx used by about 80 million patients on the global market.

It is difficult to understand how it works when a billion dollar organization decide to neutralize and discredit someone. These powers are incredibly strong. Their ways are subtle and efficient. We have already discussed how such interventions materialize. When a researcher has become the target, evil rumors and public accusations will soon start to appear, no matter how far from the truth, and his ethos and standing in the society is often ruined for good (70,216).

When the pharmaceutical industry tests a new pharmaceutical drug, the conclusion from the published documentation from the RCT is *always* that it helps, and *almost always* that it does only little harm. When the independent researchers at independent institutes use large metaanalysis and rigid protocols (the Cochrane procedures (306-308)) to test the same pharmaceutical drugs the conclusion is *sometimes* that the drugs are without positive effect at all and *often* that the drugs are dangerous and have severe adverse effects.

Most drugs do not cure, and many drugs do not even help the patients. The drugs that do help has often a ridiculously high NNT number of 50 or 100, meaning that 50 or 100 patients are to be treated for one single patient to be helped. As a principle there is no cure if you are seriously ill, physically or mentally. *The drugs cannot cure a serious disease in most cases.*

The independent researcher finds that the drugs are often just poisons that a smart industrial test-procedure, the RCT, has made look effective and harmless. Millions of sick and defenseless people trusting their doctor, who has been completely deceived and misinformed, are taking the drugs in the naïve believe that they will help them. But this is rarely the case.

Most often all the patients will get from drugs – what the cancer patients gets from the chemotherapy, the depressed gets from the antidepressant drugs, the mentally insane gets from antipsychotic drugs – is harm. Nothing but harm – and a drop of hope. Useless hope, pointless hope, silly hope. The hope that makes you take a drug that is only harming and killing you; a drug that is on the market with one single purpose: For somebody to prey on you and make money from your suffering. It cannot be any darker. This is as evil as it gets.

We find that the RCT test used by all the pharmaceutical companies today to document the effect of the chemical medicine, is scientifically invalid, and so misleading that it makes poisons look like effective and almost harmless chemical medicine.

The pharmaceutical industry who has developed this test has deluded the world; it has sold poisons as medicine and made billions of dollars, pounds and EUROS doing so.

In conclusion the randomised, clinical trial (RCT) pretends to be a double blind test against placebo. It is not. It does not test against placebo. It is not blind at all as all the patients receiving the active drug know that they are in the treatment group. The RCT does not measure on the relevant outcomes. And it does not measure in the relevant time frame.

The way the RCT test is practices it cannot do anything but make poisons look like medicine. The pharmaceutical industry had developed it in such a way that the negative, adverse effect of the drugs are hidden while the positive effects are enhanced; even if there is no positive effect at all the RCT test will still make a poisonous drug seem helpful.

The active placebo effect is used to create the illusion of a beneficial effect, and when the patient enters the toxic phase where all the negative effects are seen accumulating the measuring stops. Thus everything is turned upside down, and poisons looks just like harmless, effective medicine.

The most problematic thing is that the result of the RCT-test fraud – the effect of what we have shown there – has been known for half a century. The effect found by the pharmaceutical industry has systematically been gone in the large metaanalysis made by independent researchers. But still the pharmaceutical industry has managed to keep the drugs on the market. How did they do that? By manipulating the whole world: The researchers, scientific journals, the academic experts, the national drug improvement agencies, the physicians, and the patients.

All the many links of the chain have been manipulated; not one single link has been left untouched by the pharmaceutical industry. And this is the mastery of the manipulation: every single link has been slightly twisted; so you won't notice. But when all the links are put together they turn everything upside down because of the additive effect of the many small twists.

The thing that seems most strange is that the mismatch of the industrial result and the results of the independent researchers making test of a much higher quality: the metaanalysis – have never lead the industry to question its methods. Even more strange is it that the national agencies that have the job of controlling the industry that everybody knows need to be controlled just have given up on exercising its control.

The pharmaceutical industry have been confronted with the differences of the results but it has never taking the consequences and analyzed the RCT method in all its problematic details as we have done in this book and the paper it is based on (1).

We feel certain that every single large pharmaceutics company of the world has employed experts that know that the RCT procedure is not fair, is not scientific, and is not documenting the effects of the drugs in a reasonable and sensible way. We feel certain that these experts have told about their considerations and second thought to the company that has employed them. We feel certain that the pharmaceutics industry in general knows about the problems we have raised in this book. The way the industry and its collaborating biomedicine doctors behave towards the holistic and alternative doctors, therapist, and researchers, they obviously also know that the drugs are much less efficient that the classical methods of medicine. Why would the biomedical doctors use so much time and effort to compete, repress and destroy the holist doctors and researchers?

But this does not stop here. In every National Medicines Agency that controls the drugs there have been intelligent people with full access to the information about the problematic drugs. These people have systematically been sitting there with the info from the pharmaceutical companies and from the independent researcher, like Abel and the Cochrane researchers. They have been sufficiently trained to acknowledge the objectivity coming from independent analysis and the trustworthiness coming from the design of the metaanalysis using many studies and pooling all data from these studies, to be analyzed with much more rigid statistical methods than the pharmaceutical industry uses.

So in every national drug agency there are experts who has known this, we are absolutely sure that these people have told there bossed and their employers bout these things. Why have nothing happened, then? Easy. If you want to understand this, JUST FOLLOW THE MONEY! As always. Nothing new. As there have been so strong commercial interests in the approval and sale of the drugs, these drugs have been approved and sold. The people who benefitted form this financially simply made it p happen. This is pretty much how the capitalistic world is, is it not?

After 50 years the pharmaceutical industry has grown large. Not large in the common sense of this world. Not enormous. Not extravagantly, extremely, breathtakingly gigantic. Larger than that. Much larger. So large that hundreds of companies employing millions of people are using all their time and effort to make the manipulation and deception of the world continue, and continue at a still faster pace.

About 50% of the Danish population is chronically ill, and all these people have a free biomedical doctor, that prescribe almost everybody that enters their clinic some drugs as we have seen. The payment system is so that you get money if you see people shortly and prescribe drugs. So this is what the physicians do. They want the money. So they treat the patients accordingly. The patients are massively manipulated by thousands of hits by extremely manipulating commercials every year.

This is an easy game: The patients have bought the drugs even before coming to the doctor. This is what they want when they go there; because they have been mislead to believe that the drugs consists a solution to their health problems. This is almost never the case. But as our consciousness are easily tricked most patients never finds out that the drugs do not work. They just thing that without the drugs they would do even worse!!! Patients are week, they need to trust because they are in big troubles, and they are so easily fooled. Shame on you, Big Pharma, to exploit these week people. Shame on you to prey on the suffering, the sick and the unhappy. Shame on you to sell poisons disguised as medicine. This is a most horrible thing to do.

The power of the pharmaceutical industry lies very much in the fundamental structure of the western capitalistic society. The classical medicine, the holistic consciousness- oriented medicine, has no financial power. There is nobody who really benefits financially from a doctor talking with his patients for hours and hours, and there is nobody – no big company or boss -who makes money on the doctor using therapeutic touch.

It is quite opposite: Using this kind of medicine is just losing out an important business opportunity. Therefore the industrial medicine has completely destroyed the classical medicine in this competition. Less competent people are offering CAM treatments of little value to the patients; the valuable treatment being the holistic is represent lied about, and forgotten. This is the image of the industry, the true power manifesting itself.

The Hippocratic medicine is harmless and extremely efficient; far the most efficient kind of medicine that we know today (109,111,122,123-128,135,165, 169) (if we exclude the shamanistic tradition using hallucinogenic drugs, like the Native American medicine men using Peyote or magic mushrooms).

Pharmaceutical drugs tested with the RCT are not evidence-based. Not at all. Drugs tested with the RCT procedure are not "scientifically tested" or clinically proven" as the advertisements tells us all the time. This is not the case. Not at all. The RCT test makes poisons look like medicine. So all medicine tested with the RCT test must be suspected to be just poison.

Exceptions are drugs where you can see the effect directly on the disease, like when syphilis is cured by penicillin.

How do we test the pharmaceutical drugs?

The simple way to test the drugs is to use them on chronic patients and measure their quality of life, self-assess physical and mental health, and general ability in a number of relevant dimensions, before and after the treatment (NNT for the outcome "cured").

If the chronic patients that have not been improving for years really gets better with this treatment, the drug must be considered helpful. The chronic patients can easily serve as their own control. Randomization to the most efficient holistic medical treatment will be the most ethical study.

The acute patients are normally spontaneously cured. The body heals by itself, and drugs do rarely make a difference. Randomization to no treatment is the simplest way to document effect; randomization to the most efficient holistic medical treatment will be the most ethical study.

As the patients are not likely to be willing to participate in such experiments as they normally already has a preference for drugs or holistic non-drug treatment we doubt that the randomizations studies can be done.

A simple strategy is to compare the different treatments there are with regards to the outcome "cured", global quality of life improved, self-assess mental and physical health improved etc.

Conclusion

The pharmaceutical industry has, with its clever design of the RCT, turned everything upside down. It has deceived and mislead the whole world; it has succeeded in selling poisons as medical drugs. In doing so it has become so rich that it now is one of the most powerful entities in the modern society. It has made so much money that it has power to market any drug, and lobby any government or organization.

All the money is used to keep the power and to sell more poisonous drugs, and to influence governments and politicians, academic institutions, scientific journals, physicians and patients.

If we want this to change, we must all contribute. Half the world is chronically ill in spite of being treated with pharmaceutical drugs in spite of cures being available with holistic medicine. More and more kids and young people are filled with these poisonous drugs that only pacifies and do not improve health at all.

We need all medicine to be tested again in a way that is reliable. Until this is done we should have little faith in pharmaceutical drugs.

Chapter 13

SCIENTIFIC RÉSUMÉ

We have analyzed the pharmaceutical companies' general method for testing pharmaceutical drugs: The randomized clinical trial (RCT). We have documented that the RCT method, as it is set up and applied today by the pharmaceutical industry, has fatal errors. The RCT-method turns in its present form everything upside-down, it makes drugs that are only poisonous look like useful and harmless medicine. Thus the RCT is completely misleading.

We have identified four errors that fit together in a synergistic pattern. Together these four errors make a fatal error: The RCT method make a toxic effect appear as a beneficial effect as it works as active placebo. The toxic effect itself is by other errors of the test obscured and minimized; most importantly this is happening as a consequence of the way outcomes are measured and the timescale used for this.

The RCT-test therefore shows exactly the opposite of what it purports to show. We conclude based on our analysis of four errors in the RCT method, that it cannot be used as basis for evidence based medicine. The RCT method cannot be used to document the positive and negative effects of pharmaceutical drugs. In spite of every biomedical physician on the planet believing in it we have found that RCT simply is not a scientific procedure.

Because of the flawed RCT procedure we suspect that the chemical medicines developed based on the RCT method all are toxic and in most cases not beneficial.

REQUIREMENTS TO SECURE QUALITY OF CHEMICAL MEDICINE

To ensure the quality of pharmacological drugs all RTC-based chemical medicines must be tested again in the following way:

1) All drugs must be tested against real placebo (classic holistic-medical treatment)
2) There must use proper measure of treatment effect (global outcome measures of quality of life and health)
3) In experiments, the patients must be followed sufficiently long, at least 2 years, so that we can assess the positive and / or negative treatment effects. We recommend that the trend over time is explored (is there a decreasing effectiveness? Is there an increasing adverse reaction rate?).

4) Pharmaceutical drugs that have been tested against "no treatment" should be tested again against real placebo (classic holistic-medical care).
5) If you want to use randomization against placebo in double blind tests you should use active placebo (a substance with a similar toxic effect), with a decent measure of treatment effect (global outcome measures) and patients should also be followed here for several years. There are big ethical problems connected to this design, as the patients in the control group only will get poisons, so we cannot recommend it.
6) Positive treatment efficacy must be expressed in Number Needed to Treat (NNT) and not in horizontal risk measures. Outcomes must as a minimum always include full recovery ("cured"), self-evaluated global quality of life, self-assessed physical and mental health, and death. The NNH for each side effect should also be reported, as should the total likelihood to get an adverse effect, which is easy to determine as the combined likelihood of all negative effects together (NNHtotal). Even better this measure is included in the clinical trial.

CALL TO ACTION FOR TESTING - AND ADVICE ON FUTURE USE OF PHARMACEUTICAL DRUGS

We urge all who are involved in developing, testing, approval and use of chemical medicines: the all pharmaceutical companies, government, hospitals, doctors and all the Medical Associations, as well as the independent research centers to help documenting the chemical medicines in a fair and trustworthy way.

Until this is done, we must expect that all pharmaceutical products documented with the flawed RCT method are much more toxic and far less helpful than they appear in the product information and the drug directory. They are also much more toxic and less helpful than documented in the Cochrane metaanalyses as these are also based on the flawed RCT.

ADVICE REGARDING SPECIFIC GROUPS OF DRUGS

We find that Abel's work is done up to scientific standard and that his results must be respected. Abel's large meta-analysis (82-85) of anti-cancer chemotherapy showed a negative treatment effect on survival and quality of life for the patients treated with chemotherapy (cell poison) and he therefore strongly advised against the use of chemotherapy in the following types of cancers: colon cancer, stomach cancer, pancreas cancer, bladder cancer, breast cancer, ovarian cancer, cervical cancer and endometrial cancer; he recommended caution regarding the treatment of small cell lung cancer and non-small cell lung cancer with chemotherapy. We recommend that Abel's recommendations are followed.

As there has been found insignificant effects of antidepressants when compared with active placebo in a Cochrane analyse (132) we must advise against the use of the antidepressant drugs.

As there has been found no positive effects on mental health ("mental state") in a large Cochrane metaanalyse (133) we advise against the use of antipsychotic drugs. We also warn that these drugs may lead to poisoning with a tendency of increased spontaneous mortality (209) and possibly also drug-induced depressions (134) and increased tendency to suicide (210).

We must call for increased awareness of adverse effects and events of any pharmaceutical product, including vaccines (68,69), antibiotics 163) and pain killers (67), which have been tested and approved on the basis of the RCT method.

All these drugs are likely to be much more harmful and much less helpful than written in the product information and in the national drug directory.

ABOUT THE AUTHORS

Søren Ventegodt, MD, MMedSci, EU-MSc is the director of the independent Quality of Life Research Center in Copenhagen, and Research Clinic for Holistic Medicine and Sexology, Copenhagen. He teaches holistic medicine, psychiatry and sexology at the Nordic School of Holistic Health and Denmark. Since 2006 he has been director for and lecturer at Inter-University College, International Campus, Denmark in collaboration with Inter-University Consortium for Integrative Health Promotion, Inter-University College Graz, Austria and the Austrian Ministry of Education, Science and Culture. He is a popular speaker throughout Scandinavia with more than 1000 presentations and for the last 10 years he has taught quality of life in the Danish Army. As holistic physician he has treated over 500 chronically ill patients and given more than 10.000 hours of holistic therapy. He has published numerous scientific or popular articles and a number of books on holistic medicine, quality of life and quality of working life. He is reviewer for more than 10 scientific journals. 130 of his scientific papers on quality of life and holistic medicine are listed on www.pubmed.gov making him one of the most productive scientists in these fields. His most important scientific contributions are the theory of holistic healing, the integrated quality of life (QOL) theory, the comprehensive SEQOL questionnaire, the very short QOL5 questionnaire, the life mission theory, and the ongoing Danish Quality of Life Research Survey, 1991-94 in connection with follow-up studies of the Copenhagen Perinatal Birth Cohort 1959-61 initiated at the University Hospital of Copenhagen by the late professor of pediatrics, Bengt Zachau-Christiansen, MD, PhD. E-Mail: ventegodt@livskvalitet.org. Website: www.livskvalitet.org

Joav Merrick, MD, MMedSci, DMSc, is professor of pediatrics, child health and human development affiliated with Kentucky Children's Hospital, University of Kentucky, Lexington, United States and the Department of Pediatrics, Hadassah-Hebrew University Medical Center, Mount Scopus Campus, Jerusalem, Israel, the medical director of the Division for Mental Retardation, Ministry of Social Affairs and Social Services, Jerusalem, the founder and director of the National Institute of Child Health and Human Development. Numerous publications in the field of pediatrics, child health and human development, rehabilitation, intellectual disability, disability, health, welfare, abuse, advocacy, quality of life and prevention. Received the Peter Sabroe Child Award for outstanding work on behalf of Danish Children in 1985 and the International LEGO-Prize ("The Children's Nobel Prize") for an extraordinary contribution towards improvement in child welfare and well-being in 1987. E-mail: jmerrick@zahav.net.il; Home-page: http://jmerrick50.googlepages.com/home

About the Quality of Life Research Center in Copenhagen, Denmark

The Quality of Life Research Center in Copenhagen was established in 1989, when the physician Søren Ventegodt succeeded in getting a collaboration started with the Department of Social Medicine at the University of Copenhagen in response to the project "Quality of life and causes of disease". An interdisciplinary "Working group for the quality of life in Copenhagen" was established and when funds were raised in 1991 the University Hospital of Copenhagen (Rigshospitalet) opened its doors for the project.

The main task was a comprehensive follow-up of 9,006 pregnancies and the children delivered during 1959-61. This Copenhagen Perinatal Birth Cohort was established by the a gynecologist and a pediatrician, the late Aage Villumsen, MD, PhD and the late Bengt Zachau-Christiansen, MD, PhD, who had made intensive studies during pregnancy, early childhood and young adulthood. The cohort was during 1980-1989 directed by the pediatrician Joav Merrick, MD, DMSc, who established the Prospective Pediatric Research Unit at the University Hospital of Copenhagen and managed to update the cohort for further follow-up register research, until he moved to Israel. The focus was to study quality of life related to socio-economic status and health in order to compare with the data collected during pregnancy, deliverty and early childhood.

The project continued to grow and later in 1993, the work was organized into a statistics group, a software group that developed the computer programs for use in the data entry and a group responsible for analysis of the data.

Quality of Life Research Center at the University Medical Center

The Quality of Life Center at the University Hospital generated grants, publicity with research and discussions among the professionals leading to the claim that quality of life was significant for health and disease. It is obvious that a single person cannot do much about his/her own disease, if it is caused by chemical defects in the body or outside chemical-physical influences. However, if a substantial part of diseases are caused by a low quality of life, we can all prevent a lot of disease and operate as our own physicians, if we make a personal effort and work to improve our quality of life. A series of investigations showed that this was indeed possible. This view of the role of personal responsibility for illness and health would naturally lead to a radical re-consideration of the role of the physician and also influence our society.

INDEPENDENT QUALITY OF LIFE RESEARCH CENTER

In 1994, The Quality of Life Research Center became an independent institution located in the center of the old Copenhagen. Today, the number of full-time employees have grown. The Research Center is still expanding and several companies and numerous institutions make use of the resources, such as lectures, courses, consulting or contract research. The companies, which have used the competence of the reseach center and its tools on quality of life and quality of working life, include IBM, Lego, several banks, a number of counties, municipalities, several ministries, The National Defense Center for Leadership and many other management training institutions, along with more than 300 public and private companies. It started in Denmark, but has expanded to involve the whole Scandinavian area.

The center's research on the quality of life have been through several phases from measurement of quality of life, from theory to practice over several projects on the quality of life in Denmark, which have been published and received extended public coverage and public impact in Denmark and Scandinavia. The data is now also an important part of Veenhoven's Database on Happiness at Rotterdam University in the Netherlands.

NEW RESEARCH

Since The Quality-of-Life Research Center became independent a number of new research projects were launched. One was a project that aimed to prevent illness and social problems among the elderly in one of the municipalities by inspiring the elderly to improve their quality of life themselves. Another a project about quality of life after apoplectic attacks at one of the major hospitals in Copenhagen and the Danish Agency for Industry granted funds for a project about the quality of work life.

QUALITY OF LIFE OF 10,000 DANES

There is a general consensus that many of the diseases that plague the Western world (which are not the result of external factors such as starvation, micro-organisms, infection or genetic defects) are lifestyle related and as such, preventable through lifestyle changes. Thus increasing time and effort is spent on developing public health strategies to promote "healthy" lifestyles. However, it is not a simple task to identify and dispel the negative and unhealthy parts of our modern lifestyle even with numerous behavioural factors that can be readily highlighted harmful, like the use of alcohol, use of tobacco, the lack of regular exercise and a high fat, low fibre diet.

However there is more to Western culture and lifestyle than these factors and if we only focus on them we can risk overlooking others. We refer to other large parts of our life, for instance the way we think about and perceive life (our life attitudes, our perception of reality and our quality of life) and the degree of happiness we experience through the different dimensions of our existence. These factors or dimensions can now, to some degree, be isolated and examined. The medical sociologist Aaron Antonovsky (1923-1994) from the Faculty of Health Sciences at Ben Gurion University in Beer-Sheva, who developed the salutogenic model of health and illness, discussed the dimension, "sense of coherence", that is closely related to the dimension of "life meaning", as perhaps the deepest and most important dimension of quality of life. Typically, the clinician or researcher, when attempting to reveal a connection between health and a certain factor, sides with only one of the possible dimensions stated above. A simple, one-dimensional hypothesis is then postulated, like for instance that cholesterol is harmful to circulation. Cholesterol levels are then measured, manipulated and ensuing changes to circulatory function monitored. The subsequent result may show a significant, though small connection, which supports the initial hypothesis and in turn becomes the basis for implementing preventive measures, like a change of diet. The multi-factorial dimension is therefore often overlooked.

In order to investigate this multifactorial dimension a cross-sectional survey examining close to 10,000 Danes was undertaken in order to investigate the connection between lifestyle, quality of life and health status by way of a questionnaire based survey. The questionnaire was mailed in February 1993 to 2,460 persons aged between 18-88, randomly selected from the CPR (Danish Central Register) and 7,222 persons from the Copenhagen Perinatal Birth Cohort 1959-61.

A total of 1,501 persons between the ages 18-88 years and 4,626 persons between the ages 31-33 years returned the questionnaire (response rates 61.0% and 64,1% respectively). The results showed that health had a stronger correlation to quality of life ($r= 0.5$, $p<0.0001$), than it had to lifestyle ($r=0.2$, $p< 0.0001$).

It was concluded that preventable diseases could be more effectively handled through a concentrated effort to improve quality of life rather than through n approach that focus solely on the factors that are traditionally seen to reflect an unhealthy life style.

COLLABORATIONS ACROSS BORDERS

The project has been developed during several phases. The first phase, 1980-1990, was about mapping the medical systems of the pre-modern cultures of the world, understanding their philosophies and practices and merging this knowledge with western biomedicine. A huge task seemingly successfully accomplished in the Quality of Life (QOL) theories, and the QOL philosophy, and the most recent theories of existence, explaining the human nature, and especially the hidden resources of man, their nature, their location in human existence and the way to approach them through human consciousness.

Søren Ventegodt visited several countries around the globe in the late 1980s and analysed about 10 pre-modern medical systems and a dozen of shamans, shangomas and spiritual leaders noticing most surprisingly similarities, allowing him together with about 20 colleagues at the QOL Study Group at the University of Copenhagen, to model the connection between QOL and health. This model was later further developed and represented in the integrative QOL theories and a number of publications. Based on this philosophical breakthrough the Quality of Life Research Center was established at the University hospital. Here a brood cooperation took place with many interested physicians and nurses from the hospital.

A QOL conference in 1993 with more than 100 scientific participants discussed the connection between QOL and the development of disease and its prevention. Four physicians collaborated on the QOL population survey 1993. For the next 10 years the difficult task of integrating bio-medicine and the traditional medicine went on and Søren Ventegodt again visited several centers and scientists at the Universities of New York, Berkeley, Stanford and other institutions. He also met people like David Spiegel, Dean Ornish, Louise Hay, Dalai Lama and many other leading persons in the field of holistic medicine and spirituality.

Around the year 2000 an international scientific network started to take form with an intense collaboration with the National Institute of Child Health and Human Development (NICHD) in Israel, which has now developed the concept of "Holistic Medicine". We believe that the trained physician today has three medical toolboxes: the manual medicine (traditional), the bio-medicine (with drugs and pharmacology) and the consciousness-based medicine (scientific, holistic medicine). What is extremely interesting is that most diseases can be alleviated with all three sets of medical tools, but only the bio-medical toolset is highly expensive. The physician, using his hands and his consciousness to improve the health of the patient by mobilising hidden resources in the patient can use his skills in any cultural setting, rich or poor.

Contact person

Director Søren Ventegodt, MD, MMedSci, MSc

Quality of Life Research Center, Frederiksberg Alle 13A, 2tv, DK-1820 Copenhagen V Denmark

E-mail: ventegodt@livskvalitet.org; Website: www.livskvalitet.org

Support our research

The Quality-of-Life Research Center, Copenhagen, is a private research center, which for the last 20 years has taken international leadership in research on quality of life and holistic medicine. A large number of scientific publications many of which are listed in www.pubmed.gov, the world's most recognized medical database, has made the research center among the leading research institutes of holistic health worldwide. The research center has collected more than 6 million USD for its research making it the leading fundraiser for research in holistic medicine in Scandinavia. Through these funding we have managed to establish an international cooperation that currently involves researchers from all continents.

Research just cost a lot of money, and we need more research to be done. You can help us by giving your contribution to the Quality of Life Research Center (account with Danske Bank SWIFT: DABADKKK; IBAN: DK7330003113434252).

It is important for us that you understand that your contribution, even if it is just 10 USD, has great importance for us in this phase. Our goal is the establishment of the first major research hospital in holistic medicine.

The establishment of this research hospital is estimated to cost around 10 million dollars. It will be able to document the efficacy of scientific holistic medicine for a wide variety of patient groups, including patients with schizophrenia and cancer. A holistic-medical research hospital will also carry out comparative studies of the efficacy of biomedicine and holistic medicine for a number of diseases. It could thus generate much of the knowledge being sought for in this book.

Please visit the website www.livskvalitet.org and feel free to write to Søren Ventegodt MD, director of the research center (email: ventegodt@livskvalitet.org).

Wills for Quality of Life Research Center

We have been running for 20 years and the international research group affiliated with the research center will for the next many years continue the research. We will therefore also need continued support. We kindly encourage you to bequeath to the research center, owned by Søren Ventegodt MD (CPR 260361-0493).

If you want to do this we offer you free legal assistance for drafting of wills. Please write to Søren Ventegodt (email: ventegodt@livskvalitet.org) if you need more information on the research or if you have special requests for use of the resources you wish to bequeath, for example, that they should be earmarked for research into cancer or schizophrenia.

You are also welcome to call Soren Ventegodt at +45 33 14 11 13 to hear more about the research center's plans for future research and development.

About the National Institute of Child Health and Human Development in Israel

The National Institute of Child Health and Human Development (NICHD) in Israel was established in 1998 as a virtual institute under the auspicies of the Medical Director, Ministry of Social Affairs and Social Services in order to function as the research arm for the Office of the Medical Director. In 1998 the National Council for Child Health and Pediatrics, Ministry of Health and in 1999 the Director General and Deputy Director General of the Ministry of Health endorsed the establishment of the NICHD.

Mission

The mission of a National Institute for Child Health and Human Development in Israel is to provide an academic focal point for the scholarly interdisciplinary study of child life, health, public health, welfare, disability, rehabilitation, intellectual disability and related aspects of human development. This mission includes research, teaching, clinical work, information and public service activities in the field of child health and human development.

Service and academic activities

Over the years many activities became focused in the south of Israel due to collaboration with various professionals at the Faculty of Health Sciences (FOHS) at the Ben Gurion University of the Negev (BGU). Since 2000 an affiliation with the Zusman Child Development Center at the Pediatric Division of Soroka University Medical Center has resulted in collaboration around the establishment of the Down Syndrome Clinic at that center. In 2002 a full course on "Disability" was established at the Recanati School for Allied Professions in the Community, FOHS, BGU and in 2005 collaboration was started with the Primary Care Unit of the faculty and disability became part of the master of public health course on "Children and society". In the academic year 2005-2006 a one semester course on "Aging with disability" was started as part of the master of science program in gerontology in our collaboration with the Center for Multidisciplinary Research in Aging. From 2011 teaching second, fourth and six year medical students at Hadassah-Hebrew University Medical Center, Jerusalem.

RESEARCH ACTIVITIES

The affiliated staff have over the years published work from projects and research activities in this national and international collaboration. In the year 2000 the International Journal of Adolescent Medicine and Health and in 2005 the International Journal on Disability and Human development of Freund Publishing House (London and Tel Aviv), in the year 2003 the TSW-Child Health and Human Development and in 2006 the TSW-Holistic Health and Medicine of the Scientific World Journal (New York and Kirkkonummi, Finland), all peer-reviewed international journals were affiliated with the National Institute of Child Health and Human Development. From 2008 also the International Journal of Child Health and Human Development (Nova Science, New York), the International Journal of Child and Adolescent Health (Nova Science) and the Journal of Pain Management (Nova Science) affiliated and from 2009 the International Public Health Journal (Nova Science) and Journal of Alternative Medicine Research (Nova Science).

NATIONAL COLLABORATION

Nationally the NICHD works in collaboration with the Faculty of Health Sciences, Ben Gurion University of the Negev; Department of Physical Therapy, Sackler School of Medicine, Tel Aviv University; Autism Center, Assaf HaRofeh Medical Center; National Rett and PKU Centers at Chaim Sheba Medical Center, Tel HaShomer; Department of Physiotherapy, Haifa University; Department of Education, Bar Ilan University, Ramat Gan, Faculty of Social Sciences and Health Sciences; College of Judea and Samaria in Ariel and in 2011 affiliation with Center for Pediatric Chronic Illness and Center for Down Syndrome, Department of Pediatrics, Hadassah-Hebrew University Medical Center, Mount Scopus Campus, Jerusalem.

INTERNATIONAL COLLABORATION

Internationally with the Department of Disability and Human Development, College of Applied Health Sciences, University of Illinois at Chicago; Strong Center for Developmental Disabilities, Golisano Children's Hospital at Strong, University of Rochester School of Medicine and Dentistry, New York; Centre on Intellectual Disabilities, University of Albany, New York; Centre for Chronic Disease Prevention and Control, Health Canada, Ottawa; Chandler Medical Center and Children's Hospital, Kentucky Children's Hospital, Section of Adolescent Medicine, University of Kentucky, Lexington; Chronic Disease Prevention and Control Research Center, Baylor College of Medicine, Houston, Texas; Division of Neuroscience, Department of Psychiatry, Columbia University, New York; Institute for the

Study of Disadvantage and Disability, Atlanta; Center for Autism and Related Disorders, Department Psychiatry, Children's Hospital Boston, Boston; Department of Paediatrics, Child Health and Adolescent Medicine, Children's Hospital at Westmead, Westmead, Australia; International Centre for the Study of Occupational and Mental Health, Düsseldorf, Germany; Centre for Advanced Studies in Nursing, Department of General Practice and Primary Care, University of Aberdeen, Aberdeen, United Kingdom; Quality of Life Research Center, Copenhagen, Denmark; Nordic School of Public Health, Gottenburg, Sweden, Scandinavian Institute of Quality of Working Life, Oslo, Norway; Centre for Quality of Life of the Hong Kong Institute of Asia-Pacific Studies and School of Social Work, Chinese University, Hong Kong.

TARGETS

Our focus is on research, international collaborations, clinical work, teaching and policy in health, disability and human development and to establish the NICHD as a permanent institute in Israel in order to conduct model research and together with the four university schools of public health/medicine in Israel establish a national master and doctoral program in disability and human development at the institute to secure the next generation of professionals working in this often non-prestigious/low-status field of work. For this project we need your support. We are looking for all kinds of support and eventually an endowment.

SUPPORT FOR OUR WORK

In the United States

In the United States the Israel Foundation for Human Development was created in order to support the work of the National Institute of Child Health and Human Development in Israel. It is possible to send donations to the Israel Foundation for Human Development Inc, which is a recognized tax-exempt organization in the United States (charitable non-for-prifit organization with 501c (3) tax exempt number 56-230-6116). Checks for the Foundation in the United States can be send to Israel Foundation for Human Development Inc., President Arlene Feldman, 2 Lawrence Street, New Hyde Park, New York 11040. Phone: 516-352-3596. E-mail: AFeldman@FarrellFritz.com

Contact in Israel

Professor Joav Merrick, MD, MMedSci, DMSc
Medical Director, Division for Mental Retardation
Ministry of Social Affairs, POBox 1260
IL-91012 Jerusalem, Israel
E-mail: jmerrick@zahav.net.il

ABOUT THE BOOK SERIES "HEALTH AND HUMAN DEVELOPMENT"

Health and human development is a book series with publications from a multidisciplinary group of researchers, practitioners and clinicians for an international professional forum interested in the broad spectrum of health and human development.

- Merrick J, Omar HA, eds. Adolescent behavior research. International perspectives. New York: Nova Science, 2007.
- Kratky KW. Complementary medicine systems: Comparison and integration. New York: Nova Science, 2008.
- Schofield P, Merrick J, eds. Pain in children and youth. New York: Nova Science, 2009.
- Greydanus DE, Patel DR, Pratt HD, Calles Jr JL, eds. Behavioral pediatrics, 3 ed. New York: Nova Science, 2009.
- Ventegodt S, Merrick J, eds. Meaningful work: Research in quality of working life. New York: Nova Science, 2009.
- Omar HA, Greydanus DE, Patel DR, Merrick J, eds. Obesity and adolescence. A public health concern. New York: Nova Science, 2009.
- Lieberman A, Merrick J, eds. Poverty and children. A public health concern. New York: Nova Science, 2009.
- Goodbread J. Living on the edge. The mythical, spiritual and philosophical roots of social marginality. New York: Nova Science, 2009.
- Bennett DL, Towns S, Elliot E, Merrick J, eds. Challenges in adolescent health: An Australian perspective. New York: Nova Science, 2009.
- Schofield P, Merrick J, eds. Children and pain. New York: Nova Science, 2009.
- Sher L, Kandel I, Merrick J. Alcohol-related cognitive disorders: Research and clinical perspectives. New York: Nova Science, 2009.
- Anyanwu EC. Advances in environmental health effects of toxigenic mold and mycotoxins. New York: Nova Science, 2009.
- Bell E, Merrick J, eds. Rural child health. International aspects. New York: Nova Science, 2009.
- Dubowitz H, Merrick J, eds. International aspects of child abuse and neglect. New York: Nova Science, 2010.

- Shahtahmasebi S, Berridge D. Conceptualizing behavior: A practical guide to data analysis. New York: Nova Science, 2010.
- Wernik U. Chance action and therapy. The playful way of changing. New York: Nova Science, 2010.
- Omar HA, Greydanus DE, Patel DR, Merrick J, eds. Adolescence and chronic illness. A public health concern. New York: Nova Science, 2010.
- Patel DR, Greydanus DE, Omar HA, Merrick J, eds. Adolescence and sports. New York: Nova Science, 2010.
- Shek DTL, Ma HK, Merrick J, eds. Positive youth development: Evaluation and future directions in a Chinese context. New York: Nova Science, 2010.
- Shek DTL, Ma HK, Merrick J, eds. Positive youth development: Implementation of a youth program in a Chinese context. New York: Nova Science, 2010.
- Omar HA, Greydanus DE, Tsitsika AK, Patel DR, Merrick J, eds. Pediatric and adolescent sexuality and gynecology: Principles for the primary care clinician. New York: Nova Science, 2010.
- Chow E, Merrick J, eds. Advanced cancer. Pain and quality of life. New York: Nova Science, 2010.
- Latzer Y, Merrick, J, Stein D, eds. Understanding eating disorders. Integrating culture, psychology and biology. New York: Nova Science, 2010.
- Sahgal A, Chow E, Merrick J, eds. Bone and brain metastases: Advances in research and treatment. New York: Nova Science, 2010.
- Postolache TT, Merrick J, eds. Environment, mood disorders and suicide. New York: Nova Science, 2010.
- Maharajh HD, Merrick J, eds. Social and cultural psychiatry experience from the Caribbean Region. New York: Nova Science, 2010.
- Mirsky J. Narratives and meanings of migration. New York: Nova Science, 2010.
- Harvey PW. Self-management and the health care consumer. New York: Nova Science, 2011.
- Ventegodt S, Merrick J. Sexology from a holistic point of view. New York: Nova Science, 2011.
- Ventegodt S, Merrick J. Principles of holistic psychiatry: A textbook on holistic medicine for mental disorders. New York: Nova Science, 2011.
- Greydanus DE, Calles Jr JL, Patel DR, Nazeer A, Merrick J, eds. Clinical aspects of psychopharmacology in childhood and adolescence. New York: Nova Science, 2011.
- Bell E, Seidel BM, Merrick J, eds. Climate change and rural child health. New York: Nova Science, 2011.
- Bell E, Zimitat C, Merrick J, eds. Rural medical education: Practical strategies. New York: Nova Science, 2011.
- Latzer Y, Tzischinsky. The dance of sleeping and eating among adolescents: Normal and pathological perspectives. New York: Nova Science, 2011.

CONTACT

Professor Joav Merrick, MD, MMedSci, DMSc
Medical Director, Health Services, Division for Mental Retardation
Ministry of Social Affairs, POBox 1260
IL-91012 Jerusalem, Israel
E-mail: jmerrick@internet-zahav.net

ACKNOWLEDGMENTS

The Danish Quality of Life Survey and the Quality of Life Research Center was 1991-2004 supported by grants from the 1991 Pharmacy Foundation, the Goodwill-fonden, the JL-Foundation, E. Danielsen and Wife's Foundation, Emmerick Meyer's Trust, the Frimodt-Heineken Foundation, the Hede Nielsen Family Foundation, Petrus Andersens Fond, Wholesaler C.P. Frederiksens Study Trust, Else and Mogens Wedell-Wedellsborg's Foundation and IMK Almene Fond. The research in quality of life and scientific complementary and holistic medicine was approved by the Copenhagen Scientific Ethical Committee under the numbers (KF)V. 100.1762-90, (KF)V. 100.2123/91, (KF)V. 01-502/93, (KF)V. 01-026/97, (KF)V. 01-162/97, (KF)V. 01-198/97, and further correspondence. We declare no conflicts of interest.

REFERENCES

(1) Ventegodt S, Andersen NJ, Brom B, Merrick J, Greydanus DE. Evidence-based medicine: Four fundamental problems with the randomised clinical trial (RTC) used to document chemical medicine. Int. J. Adolesc. Med. Health 2009;21(4):484-96.

(2) Folkesundhedsrapporten Danmark 2007]. Copenhagen: Statens Inst. Folkesundhed, 2007. [Danish] [No authors listed]

(3) Jones WHS. Hippocrates. Vol. I–IV. London: William Heinemann, 1923-1931.

(4) Ventegodt S. [En teori for bevidsthedsorienteret medicin: Livsformålsteorien (life mission theory)]. Awareness-oriented (holistic) medical theory: the purpose of life theory the life mission theory)] Ugeskr Laeger 2003;165(6):590. [Danish]

(5) Ventegodt S, Andersen NJ, Merrick J. Editorial: Five theories of human existence. Scientific World Journal 2003;3:1272-6.

(6) Ventegodt S. The life mission theory: A theory for a consciousness-based medicine. Int. J. Adolesc. Med. Health 2003;15(1):89-91.

(7) Ventegodt S, Andersen NJ, Merrick J. The life mission theory II: The structure of the life purpose and the ego. Scientific World Journal 2003;3:1277-85.

(8) Ventegodt S, Andersen NJ, Merrick J. The life mission theory III: Theory of talent. Scientific World Journal 2003;3:1286-93.

(9) Ventegodt S, Merrick J. The life mission theory IV. A theory of child development. Scientific World Journal 2003;3:1294-1301.

(10) Ventegodt S, Andersen NJ, Merrick J. The life mission theory V. A theory of the anti-self and explaining the evil side of man. Scientific World Journal 2003;3:1302-13.

(11) Ventegodt S, Andersen NJ, Merrick J. The life mission theory VI: A theory for the human character. Scientific World Journal 2004;4:859-80.

(12) Ventegodt S, Flensborg-Madsen T, Andersen NJ, Merrick J. Life Mission Theory VII: Theory of existential (Antonovsky) coherence: a theory of quality of life, health and ability for use in holistic medicine. Scientific World Journal 2005;5:377-89.

(13) Ventegodt S, Merrick J. Life mission theory VIII: A theory for pain. J. Pain Manage 2008;1(1):5-10.

(14) Ventegodt S. Life mission theory IX: Integrative, ethical theory. J. Altern. Med. Res. 2009;1(3):301-12.

(15) Ventegodt S, Andersen NJ, Kandel I, Merrick J. The open source protocol of clinical holistic medicine. J. Altern. Med. Res. 2009;1(2):129-44.

(16) Ventegodt S, Merrick J. Clinical holistic medicine: Applied consciousness-based medicine. Scientific World Journal 2004;4:96-9.

(17) Ventegodt S, Flensborg-Madsen T, Andersen NJ, Nielsen M, Mohammed M, Merrick J. Global quality of life (QOL), health and ability are primarily determined by our consciousness. Research findings from Denmark 1991-2004. Soc. Indicator Res. 2005;71:87-122.

(18) Ventegodt S, Kandel I, Merrick J. Quality of life and philosophy of life determines physical and mental health: status over research findings from the Quality of Life Research Center, Copenhagen, 1991-2007. Scientific World Journal 2007;7:1743-51.

(19) Ventegodt S, Flensborg-Madsen T, Andersen NJ, Nielsen M, Morad M, Merrick J. Global quality of life (QOL), health and ability are primarily determined by our consciousness. Research findings from Denmark 1991-2004. In: Shek DTL, Chan YK, Lee PSN, eds. Quality of life research in Chinese, Western and global contexts. Dordrecht, Netherlands: Springer, 2005:87-122.
(20) Ventegodt S, Merrick J. Lifestyle, quality of life and health. Scientific World Journal 2003;3:811-25.
(21) Ventegodt S, Andersen NJ, Merrick J. Holistic Medicine II: The square-curve paradigm for research in alternative, complementary and holistic medicine: A cost-effective, easy and scientifically valid design for evidence based medicine. Scientific World Journal 2003;3:1117-27.
(22) Ventegodt S, Merrick J. Personality disorders and clinical holistic medicine. The revival of traditional holistic medicine in a modern scientific form. In: Hagen JC, Jensen EI, eds. Personality disorders: New research. New York: Nova Sci, in press.
(23) Ventegodt S, Morad M, Andersen NJ, Merrick J. Clinical holistic medicine Tools for a medical science based on consciousness. Scientific World Journal 2004;4:347-61.
(24) Ventegodt S, Clausen B, Nielsen ML, Merrick J. Advanced tools for holistic medicine. Scientific World Journal 2006;6:2048-65.
(25) Ventegodt S, Morad M, Hyam E, Merrick J. Clinical holistic medicine: When biomedicine is inadequate. Scientific World Journal 2004;4:333-46.
(26) Ventegodt S, Kandel I, Merrick J. A short history of clinical holistic medicine. Scientific World Journal 2007;7:1622-30.
(27) Ventegodt S, Kandel I, Merrick J. Biomedicine or holistic medicine for treating mentally ill patients? A philosophical and economical analysis. Scientific World Journal 2007;7:1978-86.
(28) Ventegodt S, Merrick J. What is the most efficient way to improve health: Changing your lifestyle or improving your quality of life? In: Kinger LV, ed. Focus on lifestyle and health research. New York: Nova Science, 2005;1-22.
(29) Ventegodt S, Kandel I, Merrick J. CAM is tested unfairly against placebo – CAM is offering highly efficient placebo cures that should be tested with respect for its nature. BMJ 2007 Oct 14. On-line: http://www.bmj.com/cgi/eletters/335/7623/743#178119.
(30) Ventegodt S, Andersen NJ, Kandel I, Merrick J. Formal errors in nonpharmaceutical medicine (CAM): Clinical medicine, mind-body medicine, body-psychotherapy, holistic medicine, clinical holistic medicine and sexology. Int. J. Adolesc. Med. Health 2009;21(2):161-74.
(31) Ventegodt S, Andersen NJ, Kandel I, Merrick J. Tools for comparative evaluation of the effect of drug and non-drug medical treatments. J. Altern. Med. Res. 2010;2(2):129-35.
(32) Ventegodt S. [Livskvalitet – at erobre livets mening og blive rask igen]. Quality of Life. To seize the meaning of life and become well again. Copenhagen: Forskningscentrets Forlag, 1995. [Danish]
(33) Ventegodt S. [Livsfilosofi der helbreder]. Philosophy of life that heals. Copenhagen: Forskningscenterets Forlag, 1999. [Danish]
(34) Ventegodt S. [Livskvalitet som medicin]. Quality of life as medicine Copenhagen: Forskningscenterets Forlag, 2001. [Danish]
(35) Ventegodt S. [Bevidsthedsmedicin – set gennem lægejournalen]. Consciousness-based medicine. Copenhagen: Forskningscenterets Forlag, 2003. [Danish]
(36) Ventegodt S. [Arbejdslivskvalitet - at blive værdifuld for sig selv og sin omverden]. Forskningscenterets Forlag, 1996. [Danish]
(37) Ventegodt S, Kandel I, Merrick J. Principles of holistic medicine. Philosophy behind quality of life. Victoria, BC: Trafford, 2005.
(38) Ventegodt S, Kandel I, Merrick J. Principles of holistic medicine. Quality of life and health. New York: Hippocrates Sci. Publ., 2005.
(39) Ventegodt S, Kandel I, Merrick J. Principles of holistic medicine. Global quality of life.Theory, research and methodology. New York: Hippocrates Sci. Publ., 2005.
(40) Ventegodt S. [Måling af livskvalitet. Fra teori til praksis]. Copenhagen: Forskningscentrets Forlag, 1995. [Danish]
(41) Ventegodt S. Measuring the quality of life. From theory to practice. Copenhagen: Forskningscentrets Forlag, 1996.

(42) Ventegodt S. Livskvalitet i Danmark / Quality of life in Denmark. Results from a population survey. Copenhagen: Forskningscentrets Forlag, 1995. [partly in Danish]

(43) Ventegodt S. Livskvalitet hos 4500 31-33 årige / The quality of life of 4500 31-33 year-olds. Result from a study of the Prospective Pediatric Cohort of persons born at the University Hospital in Copenhagen. Copenhagen: Forskningscentrets Forlag, 1996. [partly in Danish]

(44) Ventegodt S. Livskvalitet og omstændigheder tidligt i livet / The quality of life and factors in pregnancy, birth and infancy. Results from a follow-up study of the Prospective Pediatric Cohort of persons born at the University Hospital in Copenhagen 1959-61. Copenhagen: Forskningscentrets Forlag, 1995. [partly in Danish]

(45) Ventegodt S. Livskvalitet og livets store begivenheder / The quality of life and major events in life. Copenhagen: Forskningscentrets Forlag, 2000. [partly in Danish]

(46) Antonella R. Introduction of regulatory methods. Graz, Austria: Interuniversity College, 2004.

(47) Blättner B. Fundamentals of salutogenesis. Graz, Austria: Interuniversity College, 2004.

(48) Endler PC. Master program for complementary, psychosocial and integrated health sciences Graz, Austria: Interuniversity College, 2004.

(49) Endler PC. Working and writing scientifically in complementary medicine and integrated health sciences. Graz, Austria: Interuniversity College, 2004.

(50) Kratky KW. Complementary medicine systems. Comparison and integration. New York, Nova Sci, 2008.

(51) Pass PF. Fundamentals of depth psychology. Therapeutic relationship formation between self-awareness and casework Graz, Austria: Interuniversity College, 2004.

(52) Spranger HH. Fundamentals of regulatory biology. Paradigms and scientific backgrounds of regulatory methods Graz, Austria: Interuniversity College, 2004.

(53) Jones E. The life and works of Sigmund Freud. New York: Basic Books, 1961.

(54) Jung CG. Man and his symbols. New York: Anchor Press, 1964.

(55) Reich W. [Die Function des Orgasmus]. Köln: Kiepenheuer Witsch 1969. [German]

(56) Reich W. Character analysis. New York: Farrar Straus Giroux, 1990.

(57) Searles HF. Collected papers on Schizophrenia. Madison, CT: Int. Univ. Press, 1965:15-8.

(58) Knight RP. Preface. In: Searles HF. Collected papers on Schizophrenia. Madison, CT: Int. Univ. Press, 1965:15-8.

(59) Maines R. The technology of orgasm. Baltimore, MD: Johns Hopkins Univ Press, Baltimore, 1999.

(60) Ventegodt S. [Min brug af vaginal akupressur]. My use of vaginal acupressure. Ugeskr Laeger 2006;168(7):715-6. [Danish]

(61) Ventegodt S, Clausen B, Omar HA, Merrick J. Clinical holistic medicine: Holistic sexology and acupressure through the vagina (Hippocratic pelvic massage). Scientific World Journal 2006;6:2066-79.

(62) Ventegodt S, Clausen B, Merrick J. Clinical holistic medicine: Pilot study on the effect of vaginal acupressure (Hippocratic pelvic massage). Scientific World Journal 2006;6:2100-16.

(63) Ventegodt S, Struck P. Five tools for manual sexological examination and treatment. J. Altern. Med. Res. 2009;1(3):247-56..

(64) Ventegodt S, Merrick J. The purpose of the medical ethic of Hippocrates was efficient healing of the patient. J. Altern. Med. Res. 2010;2(2):137-42.

(65) Ventegodt S, Merrick J. Placebo explained: Consciousness causal to health. BMJ Rapid responses 2004 Oct 22. http://bmj.com/cgi/eletters/329/7472/927#80636.

(66) Boutron I, Estellat C, Guittet L, Dechartres A, Sackett DL, Hróbjartsson A, Ravaud P. Methods of blinding in reports of randomized controlled trials assessing pharmacologic treatments: a systematic review. PLoS Med 2006;3(10):e425.

(67) Gøtzsches P. Bias in double-blind trials. Dan. Med. Bull. 1990;37:329-336.

(68) Jefferson TO, Rivetti D, Rivetti A, Rudin M, Di Pietrantonj C, Demicheli V. Efficacy and effectiveness of influenza vaccines in elderly people: A systematic review. Lancet 2005;366(9492):1165-74.

(69) Demicheli V, Rivetti D, Deeks JJ, Jefferson TO. Vaccines for preventing influenza in healthy adults. Cochrane Database Syst. Rev. 2004;3:CD001269.

(70) Ventegodt S, Merrick J, Andersen NJ. Bio- and alternative medicine in conflict. Human rights protection of the alternative therapist. J. Altern. Med. Res. 2009;1(2):189-202.

(71) Jefferson T, Zarra L, Stoica L. Attenti Alle Bufale ('Beware of Red Herrings'), or, How to Make Evidence-Based Medicine Work for You. http://jrsm.rsmjournals.com/cgi/content/citation/99/12/625. Accessed 2009-10-10.

(72) Hròbjartsson A, Gøtzsche PC. Placebo interventions for all clinical conditions. Cochrane Database Syst. Rev. 2004;(3):CD003974.

(73) Singh-Manoux A, Dugravot A, Shipley MJ, Ferrie JE, Martikainen P, Goldberg M, Zins M. The association between self-rated health and mortality in different socioeconomic groups in the GAZEL cohort study. Int. J. Epidemiol. 2007;36(6):1222-8.

(74) Long MJ, McQueen DA, Bangalore VG, Schurman JR, 2nd. Using self-assessed health to predict patient outcomes after total knee replacement. Clin. Orthop. Relat. Res. 2005;434:189-92.

(75) Idler EL, Russell LB, Davis D. Survival, functional limitations, and self-rated health in the NHANES I Epidemiologic Follow-up Study, 1992. First National Health and Nutrition Examination Survey. Am. J. Epidemiol. 2000;152(9):874-83.

(76) Idler EL, Kasl S. Health perceptions and survival: do global evaluations of health status really predict mortality? J. Gerontol. 1991;46(2):S55-65.

(77) Burström B, Fredlund P. Self rated health: Is it as good a predictor of subsequent mortality among adults in lower as well as in higher social classes. J. Epidemiol. Community Health 2001;55(11):836-40.

(78) Ventegodt S, Kandel, I, Merrick, J. Holistic psychiatry: A model for holistic diagnoses and holistic treatment of mild, borderline and psychotic personality disorders. J. Altern. Med. Res. 2010;2(2):143-54.

(79) Smith R. The drugs don't work, BMJ 2003;327(7428):0-h.

(80) Ventegodt S, Andersen NJ, Kandel I, Merrick J. Effect, side effects and adverse events of non-pharmaceutical medicine. A review. Int. J. Disabil. Hum. Dev. 2009;8(3):229-37.

(81) Ventegodt S, Kandel I, Merrick J. Therapeutic value of antipsychotic drugs: A critical analysis of Cochrane meta-analyses of the therapeutic value of anti-psychotic drugs used in Denmark. J. Altern. Med. Res. 2009;1(1):59-65.

(82) Abel U. Chemotherapy of advanced epithelial cancer - a critical review. Biomed. Pharmacother. 1992;46:439-52.

(83) Abel U. [Chemotherapy of advanced epithelial cancer.] Stuttgart: Hippokrates Verlag 1990. [German]

(84) Abel U. [Chemotherapie fortgeschrittener Karzi-nome. Eine kritische Bestandsaufnahme.] Berlin: Hippokrates, 1995. [German]

(85) Abel U. Chemotherapy of advanced epithelial cancer. Stuttgrat, Germany: Hippokrates Verlag, 1995.

(86) Ventegodt S, Endler PC, Andersen NJ, Svanberg BØ, Struve F, and Merrick J. Therapeutic value of anti-cancer drugs: A critical analysis of Cochrane meta-analyses of the therapeutic value of chemotherapy for cancer. J. Altern. Med. Res., in press.

(87) Hermansen TD, Ventegodt S, Rald E, Clausen B, Nielsen ML, Merrick J. Human development I: twenty fundamental problems of biology, medicine, and neuro-psychology related to biological information. Scientific World Journal 2006;6:747-59.

(88) Ventegodt S, Hermansen TD, Nielsen ML, Clausen B, Merrick J. Human development II: we need an integrated theory for matter, life and consciousness to understand life and healing. Scientific World Journal 2006;6:760-6.

(89) Ventegodt S, Hermansen TD, Rald E, Flensborg-Madsen T, Nielsen ML, Clausen B, Merrick J. Human development III: bridging brain-mind and body-mind. Introduction to "deep" (fractal, poly-ray) cosmology. Scientific World Journal 2006;6:767-76.

(90) Ventegodt S, Hermansen TD, Flensborg-Madsen T, Nielsen ML, Clausen B, Merrick J. Human development IV: the living cell has information-directed self-organisation. Scientific World Journal 2006;6:1132-8.

(91) Ventegodt S, Hermansen TD, Flensborg-Madsen T, Nielsen ML, Clausen B, Merrick J. Human development V: biochemistry unable to explain the emergence of biological form (morphogenesis) and therefore a new principle as source of biological information is needed. Scientific World Journal 2006;6:1359-67.

(92) Ventegodt S, Hermansen TD, Flensborg-Madsen T, Nielsen M, Merrick J. Human development VI: Supracellular morphogenesis. The origin of biological and cellular order. Scientific World Journal 2006;6:1424-33.

(93) Ventegodt S, Hermansen TD, Flensborg-Madsen T, Rald E, Nielsen ML, Merrick J. Human development VII: A spiral fractal model of fine structure of physical energy could explain central aspects of biological information, biological organization and biological creativity. Scientific World Journal 2006;6:1434-40.

(94) Ventegodt S, Hermansen TD, Flensborg-Madsen T, Nielsen ML, Merrick J. Human development VIII: A theory of "deep" quantum chemistry and cell consciousness: Quantum chemistry controls genes and biochemistry to give cells and higher organisms consciousness and complex behavior. Scientific World Journal 2006;6:1441-53.

(95) Ventegodt S, Hermansen TD, Flensborg-Madsen T, Rald E, Nielsen ML, Merrick J. Human development IX: A model of the wholeness of man, his consciousness and collective consciousness. Scientific World Journal 2006;6:1454-9.

(96) Hermansen TD, Ventegodt S, Merrick J. Human development X: Explanation of macroevolution — top-down evolution materializes consciousness. The origin of metamorphosis. Scientific World Journal 2006;6:1656-66.

(97) Hermansen TD, Ventegodt S, Kandel I. Human development XI: the structure of the cerebral cortex. Are there really modules in the brain? Scientific World Journal 2007;7:1922-9.

(98) Ventegodt S, Hermansen TD, Kandel I, Merrick J. Human development XII: a theory for the structure and function of the human brain. Scientific World Journal 2008;8:621-42.

(99) Ventegodt S, Hermansen TD, Kandel I, Merrick J. Human development XIII: the connection between the structure of the overtone system and the tone language of music. Some implications for our understanding of the human brain. Scientific World Journal 2008;8:643-57.

(100) Ventegodt S, Hermansen TD, Kandel I, Merrick J. Human development XIV: Degeneration and regeneration of existence. Metamorphosis changes the purpose of life, the level of existential responsibility, and the depth of consciousness (the ray-number of the cosmology). J. Altern. Med. Res. 2009;1(4):409-18.

(101) Ventegodt S, Hermansen TD, Kandel I, Merrick J. Human development XV: The biochemical hypothesis for the etiology of the mental diseases is not substantiated. J. Altern. Med. Res. 2009;1(4):419-32.

(102) Ventegodt S, Hermansen TD, Kandel I, Merrick J. Human development XVI: General etiology of mental diseases and the role of re-metamorphosis in spontaneous recovery ("Monster theory"). J. Altern. Med. Res. 2009;1(4):433-8.

(103) Ventegodt S, Hermansen TD, Kandel I, Merrick J. Human development XVII: Jerne's anti-idiotypic network theory cannot explain self-nonself discrimination J. Altern. Med. Res. 2009;1(4):439-44.

(104) Ventegodt S, Hermansen TD, Kandel I, Merrick J. Human development XVIII: A theory for immune system regulation (the "self-nonself discrimination"). J. Altern. Med. Res. 2009;1(4):445-52.

(105) Ventegodt S, Hermansen TD, Kandel I, Merrick J. Human development XIX: The aetiology of somatic diseases. The reason for the energetic chrisis of patients in accelerated personal growth. J. Altern. Med. Res. 2009;1(4):453-64.

(106) Ventegodt S, Hermansen TD, Kandel I, Merrick J. Human development XX: A theory for accelerated, spontaneous existential healing (salutogenesis): Adult human metamorphosis. J. Altern. Med. Res. 2009;1(4):465-74.

(107) Hermansen TD, Ventegodt S, Kandel I, Merrick J. Human development XXI: How the fly got its wings. The "fly-wing theory" explains how top down evolution gave the fly its wings, and how the Self's intent materializes biological order and body-form during fylogenesis and ontogenesis (metamorphosis). J. Altern. Med. Res. 2009;1(4):475-80.

(108) Hermansen TD, Ventegodt S, Kandel I, Merrick J. Human development XXII: Antonovsky salutogenesis induced by holistic therapy gives spontaneous recovery. Salutogenesis might be controlled by the human genes for metamorphosis. If such genes are controlled by our (sub)consciousness this could explain the large and well known placebo effect. J. Altern. Med. Res. 2009;1(4):481-90.
(109) Ventegodt S, Merrick J. Metaanalysis of positive effects, side effects, and adverse events of holistic mind-body medicine, subtype holistic, clinical medicine: "clinical holistic medicine" (Denmark, Israel) "mindful mind-body medicine" (Sweden), "biodynamic body psychotherapy" (UK), and "biodynamishe körperpsychotherapie"(Germany). A review. Int. J. Disabil. Hum. Dev. 2009, in press.
(110) Ventegodt S, Andersen NJ, Merrick J, Greydanus DE. Effectiveness of traditional pharmaceutical biomedicine versus complementary and alternative medicine in a physician's general practice. J. Altern. Med. Res. 2010;2(2):179-86.
(111) Ventegodt S, Omar HA, Merrick J. Quality of life as medicine: Interventions that induce salutogenesis. A review of the literature. Soc. indicators Res. 2011;100:415-33.
(112) Ventegodt S, Thegler S, Andreasen T, Struve F, Enevoldsen L, Bassaine L, Torp M, Merrick J. Clinical holistic medicine (mindful, short-term psychodynamic psychotherapy complemented with bodywork) in the treatment of experienced physical illness and chronic pain. Scientific World Journal 2007;7:310-6.
(113) Ventegodt S, Thegler S, Andreasen T, Struve F, Enevoldsen L, Bassaine L, Torp M, Merrick J. Clinical holistic medicine (mindful, short-term psychodynamic psychotherapy complemented with bodywork) in the treatment of experienced mental illness. Scientific World Journal 2007;7:306-9.
(114) Ventegodt S, Thegler S, Andreasen T, Struve F, Enevoldsen L, Bassaine L, Torp M, Merrick J. Clinical holistic medicine (mindful, short-term psychodynamic psychotherapy complemented with bodywork) in the treatment of experienced impaired sexual functioning. Scientific World Journal 2007;7:324-9.
(115) Ventegodt S, Thegler S, Andreasen T, Struve F, Enevoldsen L, Bassaine L, Torp M, Merrick J. Clinical holistic medicine (mindful, short-term psychodynamic psychotherapy complemented with bodywork) improves quality of life, health, and ability by induction of Antonovsky-salutogenesis. Scientific World Journal 2007;7:317-23.
(116) Ventegodt S, Thegler S, Andreasen T, Struve F, Enevoldsen L, Bassaine L, Torp M, Merrick J. Self-reported low self-esteem. Intervention and follow-up in a clinical setting. Scientific World Journal 2007;7:299-305.
(117) Ventegodt S, Andersen NJ, Merrick J. Clinical holistic medicine in the recovery of working ability. A study using Antonovsky salutogenesis. Int. J. Disabil. Hum. Dev. 2008;7(2):219-22.
(118) Ornish D, Brown SE, Scherwitz LW, Billings JH, Armstrong WT, et al. Can lifestyle changes reverse coronary heart disease? The lifestyle heart trial. Lancet 1990;336(8708), 129-33.
(119) Ornish D, Scherwitz LW, Billings JH, Brown SE, Gould KL, et al. Intensive lifestyle changes for reversal of coronary heart disease. JAMA 1998;280(23),2001-7.
(120) Krishnamani MN..From doubt to certainty. New Delhi: Rajan Publications, 2006.
(121) Spiegel D, Bloom JR, Kraemer HC, Gottheil E. Effect of psychosocial treatment on survival of patients with metastatic breast cancer. Lancet 1989;2(8668):888-91.
(122) Ventegodt S, Merrick J. A Review of Side Effects and Adverse Events of Non-Drug Medicine (Nonpharmaceutical Complementary and Alternative Medicine): Psychotherapy, Mind-Body Medicine and Clinical Holistic Medicine. J. Complement. Integr. Med., 2009,6(1):1-29.
(123) Sobel DS. Mind matters, money matters: The cost-effectiveness of mind/body medicine. JAMA 2000;284(13):1704.
(124) Sobel DS. The cost-effectiveness of mind-body medicine interventions. In: Mayer EA, Saber CB, eds. The biological basis for mind body interactions. Progr. Brain Res. 2000;122:393-412.
(125) Astin JA, Shapiro SL, Eisenberg DM, Forys KL. Mind-body medicine: State of the science. Implications for practice. J. Am. Board Fam. Pract. 2003;16:131-47.
(126) Harrington A. The cure within: a history of mind-body medicine. New York: WW Norton, 2008.
(127) Goleman D, Gurin J, Connellan H. Mind, body medicine: How to use your mind for better health. New York: Consumer Reports Books, 1993.

(128) Vickers A, Zollman C. ABC of complementary medicine. Massage therapies. BMJ 1999;319(7219):1254-7.
(129) de Vibe M, Bell E, Merrick J, Omar HA, Ventegodt S. Ethics and holistic healthcare practice. Int. J. Child Health Human Dev. 2008;1(1):23-8.
(130) Ventegodt S, Kandel I, Merrick J. First do no harm: an analysis of the risk aspects and side effects of clinical holistic medicine compared with standard psychiatric biomedical treatment. Scientific World Journal 2007;7:1810-20.
(131) Kaptchuk TJ, Kelley JM, Conboy LA, Davis RB, Kerr CE, Jacobson EE, Kirsch I, Schyner RN, Nam BH, Nguyen LT, Park M, Rivers AL, McManus C, Kokkotou E, Drossman DA, Goldman P, Lembo AJ. Components of placebo effect: randomised controlled trial in patients with irritable bowel syndrome. BMJ 2008;336(7651):999-1003.
(132) Moncrieff J, Wessely S, Hardy R. Active placebos versus antidepressants for depression. Cochrane Database Syst. Rev. 2004;(1):CD003012.
(133) Adams CE, Awad G, Rathbone J, Thornley B. Chlorpromazine versus placebo for schizophrenia. Cochrane Database Syst. Rev. 2007;(2):CD000284.
(134) SBU-rapport nr. 133/1 og 133/2. Behandling med neuroleptika. Stockholm: Statens beredning för utvärdering av medicinsk metodik, 1997. [Swedish]
(135) Ventegodt S, Andersen NJ, Kandel I, Merrick J. The effect of antipsychotic drugs and non-drug therapy on borderline and psychotic mentally ill patient's quality-adjusted life-years (QALY). J. Altern. Med. Res. 2009;1(2):205-10.
(136) Ventegodt S, Andersen NJ, Kandel I. An ethical analysis of contemporary use of coercive persuasion ("brainwashing", "mind control") in psychiatry. J. Altern. Med. Res. 2009;1(2):177-88.
(137) Fitzpatrick R, Davey C, Buxton MJ, Jones DR. Evaluating patient-based outcome measures for use in clinical trials. Health Technol. Assess 1998;14 (2):1-80.
(138) Lindholt JS, Ventegodt S, Henneberg EW. Development and validation of QoL5 for clinical databases. A short, global and generic questionnaire based on an integrated theory of the quality of life. Eur. J. Surg. 2002;168:103-7.
(139) Ventegodt S, Andersen NJ, Kandel I, Merrick J. QOL10 for clinical quality-assurance and research in treatment-efficacy: Ten key questions for measuring the global quality of life, self-rated physical and mental health, and self-rated social-, sexual- and working ability. J Altern Med Res 2009;1(2):113-22.
(140) Ventegodt S, Henneberg EW, Merrick J, Lindholt JS. Validation of two global and generic quality of life questionnaires for population screening: SCREENQOL and SEQOL. ScientificWorldJournal 2003;3:412-21.
(141) McDowell IW, Newell C. Measuring health, a guide to rating scales and quesionnaires, Oxford University Press, Oxford, 1987.
(142) van Knippenberg FCE, de Haes JCJM. Measuring the quality of life of cancer patients: psychometric properties of instruments. J. Clin. Epidemiol. 1988; 41: 1043-53.
(143) Ventafridda V, van Dam FSAM, Yancik R, Tamburine M. Assessment of quality of life and cancer treatment. Amsterdam: Excerpta Medica, 1986.
(144) Hunt SM, McKenna SP, McEwen J,Wiliams J, Papp E. The Nottingham Health Profile: subjective Health Status and Medical Consultations. Soc. Sci. Med. 1981;15:221-0.
(145) Kaasa S. Measurement of quality of life in clinical trials. Oncology 1988;49:288-94.
(146) Fitzpatrick R., Fletcher A.E., Gore S., Jones D., Spiegelhaler D., Cox D. Quality of life measures in health care. I: Applications and issues in assessment. BMJ 1992;305:1074-7.
(147) Ventegodt S, Merrick J, Andersen NJ. Editorial-A new method for generic measuring of the global quality of life. Scientific World Journal 2003;3:946-9.
(148) Ventegodt S, Hilden J, Merrick J. Measurement of quality of life I: A Methodological Framework. Scientific World Journal 2003;3:950-61.
(149) Ventegodt S, Merrick J, Andersen NJ. Measurement of quality of life II. From philosophy of life to science. Scientific World Journal 2003;3:962-71.
(150) Ventegodt S, Merrick J, Andersen NJ. Measurement of quality of life III: From the IQOL theory to the global, generic SEQOL questionnaire. Scientific World Journal 2003;3:972-91.

(151) Ventegodt S, Merrick J, Andersen NJ. Measurement of quality of life IV: Use of the SEQOL, QOL5, QOL1 and other global and generic questionnaires. Scientific World Journal 2003;3:992-1001.

(152) Ventegodt S, Merrick J, Andersen NJ. Measurement of quality of life V: How to use the SEQOL, QOL5, QOL1 and other and generic questionnaires for research. Scientific World Journal 2003;3:1002-14.

(153) Ventegodt S, Merrick J, Andersen NJ. Measurement of quality of life VI: Quality-adjusted life years (QALY) is an unfortunate use of quality of life concept. Scientific World Journal 2003;3:1015-9.

(154) Ventegodt S, Merrick J. Measurement of quality of life VII: Statistical covariation and global quality of life data. The method of weight-modified linear regression. Scientific World Journal 2003;3:1020-9.

(155) Antonovsky A. Health, stress and coping. London: Jossey-Bass, 1985.

(156) Antonovsky A. Unravelling the mystery of health. How people manage stress and stay well. San Francisco: Jossey-Bass, 1987.

(157) Rout, M. Vioxx maker Merck and Co drew up doctor hit list. April 01, 2009 http://www.theaustralian.news.com.au/story/0,25197,25272600-2702,00.html. Accessed 2009-05-11.

(158) Sikich L, Frazier JA, McClellan J, Findling RL, Vitiello B, Ritz L, et al. Double-blind comparison of first- and second-generation antipsychotics in early-onset schizophrenia and schizo-affective disorder: Findings from the treatment of early-onset schizophrenia spectrum disorders (TEOSS) study. Am. J. Psychiatry 2008; 165:1420-31.

(159) Ventegodt S, Andersen NJ, Merrick J, Greydanus DE. The best health care model: Can we learn from the Danish experience? Int. J. Disabil. Hum. Dev. 2009;8(3):237-242.

(160) Danish Parliament. Report from the Technology Council on alternative treatment. Christiansborg: Danish Parliement, 19 March 2002. [Danish]

(161) Eisenberg, DM, Davis RB, Ettner SL. Trends in alternative medicine use in the United States 1990-1997. JAMA 1998;280:1569-75.

(162) Eisenberg DM, et al. Unconventional medicine in the United States. Prevalence, costs, and patterns of use. N. Engl. J. Med. 1993;328(4):246-52.

(163) Glasziou PP, Del Mar CB, Sanders SL, Hayem M. Antibiotics for acute otitis media in children. Cochrane Database Syst. Rev. 2004;(1):CD000219.

(164) Ventegodt S, Andersen NJ, Kandel I, Merrick J. Clinical medicine and psychodynamic psychotherapy. Evaluation of the patient before intervention. J. Altern. Med. Res. 2009;1(3):313-8.

(165) Ventegodt S, Andersen NJ, Kandel I, Merrick, J. Comparative analysis of cost-effectiveness of non-drug medicine (non-pharmaceutical holistic, complementary and alternative medicine/CAM) and biomedicine (pharmaceutical drugs) for all clinical conditions. Int. J. Disabil. Hum. Dev. 2009;8(3):245-260.

(166) Ventegodt, S., Morad, M., Kandel, I., and Merrick, J. (2004) Clinical holistic medicine: Social problems disguised as illness. Scientific World Journal 4, 286-294.

(167) Ventegodt S, Morad M, Hyam E, Merrick J. Clinical holistic medicine: Use and limitations of the biomedical paradigm. Scientific World Journal 2004;4:295-306.

(168) Ventegodt S, Morad M, Merrick J. Clinical holistic medicine: Classic art of healing or the therapeutic touch. Scientific World Journal 2004;4:134-47.

(169) VentegodtS, Andersen NJ, Kandel I, Merrick J. Cost-effectiveness of non-drug medicine (complementary and alternative medicine/CAM) and pharmaceutical biomedicine (drugs) for all clinical conditions - a review using the QALY measure. In press.

(170) Susan M. Review shows no evidence that individualised herbal treatments are effective. BMJ 2007;335:743.

(171) Anderson EF. Peyote. The divine cactus. Tucson, AZ: Univ Arizona Press, 1996.

(172) Bruhn JG, de Smet PA, El-Seedi HR, Beck O. Mescaline use for 5700 years. Lancet 2002; 359(9320):1866.

(173) Mumey N. The peyote ceremony among the American Indians. Bull. Med. Libr. Assoc. 1951;39 (3):182-8.

(174) Luna LE, White, S. Ayahuaasca Reader. Santa Fe, NM: Synergetic Press, 2000.

(175) Grof S. LSD psychotherapy: Exploring the frontiers of the hidden mind. Alameda, CA: Hunter House, 1980.

(176) Leary T, Metzner R, Alpert R. The psychedelic experience. A manual based on the Tibetan book of the dead. London: Acad Press, 1969.

(177) Castaneda C. The teachings of Don Juan: A Yaqui way of knowledge. New York: Harper Collins, 1968.

(178) Huxley A. The perennial philosophy. New York: Harper Collins, 1972.

(179) Legge J. The I Ching. The book of changes. Mineala, NY: Dover Publications, 1975.

(180) Sambhava P, Thurman RA, Pa KG. The Tibetan book of the dead. New York: Bantam, 1994.

(181) Saint-Exupéry AMR. The little prince. New York: Harcourt Brace, 1943.

(182) Gunnersen SJ. Statistical yearbook 2007. Copenhagen: Danmarks Statistik, 2008.

(183) Abel U. Personal communication, 2007.

(184) http://www.kwakzalverij.nl/1101/De_Germanische_Neue_Medizin_van_Ryke_Geerd_Hamer.

(185) Ventegodt S, Andersen NJ, Merrick J. Rationality and irrationality in Ryke Geerd Hamer's System for holistic treatment of metastatic cancer. Scientific World Journal 2005;5:93–102.

(186) Ventegodt S, Andersen NJ, Kandel I and Merrick J. Rationality and irrationality in Ryke Geerd Hamer's system for treatment of metastatic cancer revisited. 2009, 1(1): 47-58.

(187) Spiegel D, Butler LD, Giese-Davis J, Koopman C, Miller E, DiMiceli S, et al. Effects of supportive-expressive group therapy on survival of patients with metastatic breast cancer: A randomized prospective trial. Cancer 2007;110(5): 1130-8.

(188) www.humlegaarden.com, accessed 2009-10-11.

(189) Andersen FS. Personal communication, 2009.

(190) Ventegodt S, Morad M, Merrick J. Clinical holistic medicine: Induction of Spontaneous Remission of Cancer by Recovery of the Human Character and the Purpose of Life (the Life Mission). Scientific World Journal 2004;4:362-77.

(191) Ventegodt S, Solheim E, Saunte ME, Morad M, Kandel I, Merrick J. Clinical holistic medicine: Metastatic cancer. Scientific World Journal 2004;4:913-35.3.

(192) Ventegodt S, Jacobsen S, Merrick J. A case of induced spontaneous remission in a patient with non-Hodgkin B-Lymphoma. J. Altern. Med. Res. 2009;1(1):101-10.

(193) Lægebog for sykepleiere. Oslo: Fabritius Sønners Forlag, 1960:42.

(194) Weiner DB. The clinical training of doctors. An essay from 1793 by Philippe Pinel. Henry E Sigerist Suppl. Bull. Hist. Med. 1980;3:1-102.

(195) Modestin J, Huber A, Satirli E, Malti T, Hell D. Long-term course of schizophrenic illness: Bleuler's study reconsidered. Am. J. Psychiatry 2003;160(12):2202-8.

(196) Knight RP. Preface. In: Searles HF. Collected papers on schizophrenia. Madison, CT: Int Univ Press, 1965:15-8.

(197) Karon BP, VandenBos G. Psychotherapy of schizophrenia. The treatment of choise. New York: Jason Aronson, 1981.

(198) Ventegodt S, Andersen NJ, Neikrug S, Kandel I, Merrick J. Clinical holistic medicine: Mental disorders in a holistic perspective. Scientific World Journal 2005;5:313-23.

(199) Ventegodt S, Andersen NJ, Neikrug S, Kandel I, Merrick J. Clinical Holistic Medicine: Holistic Treatment of Mental Disorders. Scientific World Journal 2005;5:427-45.

(200) Ventegodt S, Kandel I, Merrick J. Clinical holistic medicine (mindful short-term psychodynamic psychotherapy complimented with bodywork) in the treatment of schizophrenia (ICD10-F20/DSM-IV Code 295) and other psychotic mental diseases. Scientific World Journal 2007;7:1987-2008.

(201) Struve F. Clinical holistic medicine: Psychodynamic short-time therapy complemented with bodywork. A clinical follow-up study of 109 patients. Dissertation. Graz: Interuniversity College, 2008.

(202) Torp M. Clinical holistic medicine (mindful, short-term psychodynamic psychotherapy complemented with bodywork) in the treatment of experienced impaired sexual functioning. Dissertation. Graz: Interuniversity College, 2008.

(203) Thegler S. Clinical holistic medicine (mindful, short-term psychodynamic psychotherapy complemented with bodywork) improves quality of life, health, and ability by induction of Antonovsky-salutogenesis. Dissertation. Graz: Interuniversity College, 2008.
(204) Andresen T. Clinical holistic medicine (mindful, short-term psychodynamic psychotherapy complemented with bodywork) in the treatment of experienced physical illness and chronic pain. Dissertation. Graz: Interuniversity College, 2008.
(205) Jacobsen S. Clinical holistic medicine (mindful, short-term psychodynamic psychotherapy complemented with bodywork) in the treatment of experienced mental illness. Dissertation. Graz: Interuniversity College, 2008.
(206) Enevoldsen L. Self-reported low self-esteem. Intervention and follow-up in a clinical setting. Dissertation. Graz: Interuniversity College, 2008.
(207) Ægidius H. A review and integrative analyses of ancient holistic character medicine systems. Dissertation. Graz: Interuniversity College, 2008.
(208) Nielsen ML. Advanced tools for holistic medicine. Dissertation. Graz: Interuniversity College, 2008.
(209) Lindhardt A, ed. The use of antipsychotic drugs among the 18-64 year old patients with schizophrenia, mania, or bipolar affective disorder. Copenhagen: National Board Health, 2006. [Danish]
(210) Qin P, Nordentoft M. Suicide risk in relation to psychiatric hospitalization: evidence based on longitudinal registers. Arch. Gen. Psychiatry 2005;62(4):427-32.
(211) Hemmingsen R, Parnas, J., Gjerris, A, Reisby, N. og Kragh-Sørensen, P. Klinisk Psykiatri. 2. udg. København: Munksgaard, 2000.
(212) Petersen A. Danske medicinalfirmaer lobbyer kraftigt i USA. Dagens Medicin, Forsiden, 23-10-2009. http://www.dagensmedicin.dk/nyheder/2009/10/23/dansk-medicinalindustri-me/index.xml.
(213) Hemmingsen MA. Medicinalproducenterne Lægemiddelstyrelsen revser medicinalproducenter for ulovlig reklame. GlaxoSmithKline og Pfizer har fået besked på at trække to reklamer for deres medicin tilbage. Reklamerne var ulovlige, vurderer Lægemiddelstyrelsen. Dagens Medicin 02-06-2009. http://www.dagensmedicin.dk/nyheder/2009/06/02/laegemiddelstyrelsen-revse/index.xml.
(214) Ventegodt S, Thegler S, Andreasen T, Struve F, Jacobsen S, Torp M, Ægedius H, Enevoldsen L, Merrick J. A review and integrative analysis of ancient holistic character medicine systems. Scientific World Journal 2007;7:1821-31.
(215) Jefferson T. Personal communication, 2008.
(216) Carter JP. Racketeering in medicine. The suppression of alternatives. Norfolk, VA: Hampton Roads Publ., 1993.
(217) www.bolenreport.net/feature_articles Accessed 2008-11-04.
(218) Illich I. Limits to medicine. Medical nemesis. The expropriation of health. London: Marion Boyars, 2001.
(219) Whitaker R. Mad in America. New York: Basic Books, 2002.
(220) Lanctôt G. The medical mafia: How to get out of it alive and take back our health and wealth. Quebec: Self published, 2002.
(221) Schafer J. The trial of the medical mafia. Quebec: Voici La Clef, 1998.
(222) Wohl S. The medical industrial complex. New York: Harmony Books Crown, 1984.
(223) Park A. America's health checkup: The sorry state of American health. Time 2008 Dec 1:41-51.
(224) Null G, Dean C, Feldman M, Rasio D, Smith D. (2006) Modern healthcare system is leading cause of death. Available at" www or http//:domgill. googlepages.com/iatrogenicbyGaryNulletal.doc. Accessed 08 Feb 2009.
(225) Interuniversity, Graz, Austria. Accessed 2009 Mar 01. http://www.piaa.gov.lv/admin/files /projektu_apraksti/12_abstract_complementary_health.pdf.
(226) Miriam S. Wetzel; David M. Eisenberg; Ted J. Kaptchuk. Medicine at US Medical Schools. Courses Involving Complementary and Alternative Medicine. JAMA 1998;280(9):784-7.
(227) Ventegodt S, Morad M, Merrick J. Clinical holistic medicine: The "new medicine", the multiparadigmatic physician and the medical record. Scientific World Journal 2004;4:273-85.
(228) Deleted as the professor asked that his name was not mentioned in this book.
(229) Moore RA, Edwards JE, McQuay HJ. Sildenafil (Viagra) for male erectile dysfunction: a meta-analysis of clinical trial reports. BMC Urol. 2002 May 22;2:6.

(230) Flensborg-Madsen T, Ventegodt S, Merrick J. Sense of coherence and physical health. A review of previous findings. Scientific World Journal 2005;5:665-73.

(231) Flensborg-Madsen T, Ventegodt S, Merrick J. Why is Antonovsly's sense of coherence not correlated to physical health? Analysing Antonovsky's 29-item sense of coherence scale (SOC-29). Scientific World Journal 2005;5:767-76.

(232) Flensborg-Madsen T, Ventegodt S, Merrick J. Sense of coherence and health. The construction of an amendment to Antonovsky's sense of coherence scale (SOC II). Scientific World Journal 2006;6:2133-9.

(233) Flensborg-Madsen T, Ventegodt S, Merrick J. Sense of coherence and physical health. A cross-sectional study using a new scale (SOC II). Scientific World Journal 2006;6:2200-11.

(234) Flensborg-Madsen T, Ventegodt S, Merrick J. Sense of coherence and physical health. Testing Antonovsky's theory. Scientific World Journal 2006;6:2212-9.

(235) Flensborg-Madsen T, Ventegodt S, Merrick J. Sense of coherence and physical health. The emotional sense of coherence (SOC-E) was found to be the best-known predictor of physical health. Scientific World Journal 2006;6:2147-57.

(236) DR senior editor Torben Smidt Hansen, personal communication, 2008.

(237) Gøtzsche PC, Liberati A, Torri V, Rossetti L. Beware of surrogate outcome measures. Int. J. Technol. Assess Health Care 1996;12(2):238-46.

(238) Ventegodt S, Merrick, J. Mechanical and holistic paradigms in sexology: Viagra® represents a mechanical worldview and may cause female sexual pain. J. Pain Manage 2009;2(2):77-88.

(239) Tiefer, L. Sexology and the pharmaceutical industry: the threat of co-optation. J. Sex Research 2000;37:273-83.

(240) Masters WH, Johnson VE. Human sexual inadequacy. Philadelphia, PA: Lippincott Williams Wilkins, 1966.

(241) http://www.kcl.ac.uk/news/news_details.php?news_id=1205andyear=2009 Accessed 2009-12-16.

(242) Schor S, Karten I. Statisticall evaluation of medical journal manuscripts. Jama 1966;195:145-150.

(243) Ventegodt S, Merrick J. Lifestyle, quality of life, and health. ScientificWorldJournal 2003;3:811-25.

(244) Ventegodt S, Merrick J, Andersen NJ, Bendix T. A combination of gestalt therapy, Rosen body work, and cranio sacral herapy did not help in Chronic Whiplash-Associated Disorders (WAD). Results of a randomized clinical trial. Scientific World Journal 2004;4:1055-68.

(245) Dige U. Cancer miracles. Århus: Forlaget Hovedland, 2000. [Danish]

(246) Kugelman A, Inbar-Sanado E, Shinwell ES, Makhoul IR, Leshem M, et al. Iatrogenesis in neonatal intensive care units: Observational and interventional, prospective, multicenter study. Pediatrics 2008;122: 550-555.

(247) Kaldjian LC, Jones EW, Wu BJ, Forman-Hoffman VL, Levi BH, Rosenthal GE. Reporting medical errors to improve patient safety: A survey of physicians in teaching hospitals. Arch Intern Med 2008;168:40-6.

(248) Sari AB-A, Sheldon TA, Cracknell A, Turnbull A, Dobson Y, Grant C, et al. Extent, nature and consequences of adverse events: results of a retrospective casenote review in a large NHS hospital. Qual Saf Health Care 2007;16:434-9.

(249) Murphy JG, Stee L, McEvoy MT, Oshiro J. Journal reporting of medical errors: The wisdom of Solomon, the bravery of Achilles, and the foolishness of Pan. Chest 2007;131: 890-6.

(250) Kaji AH, Gausche-Hill M, Conrad H, Young KD, Koenig WJ, Dorsey E, Lewis RJ. Emergency medical services system changes reduce pediatric epinephrine dosing errors in the prehospital setting. Pediatrics 2006;118:1493-1500.

(251) Stelfox HT, Palmisani S, Scurlock C, Orav EJ, Bates DW. The "to err is human" report and the patient safety literature.. Qual. Saf. Health Care 2006;15:174-8.

(252) Jimenez-Corona M-E, Ponce-de-Leon-Rosales S, Rangel-Frausto S, Mohar-Betancourt A. Epidemiology of medical complaints in Mexico: identifying a general profile. Int. J. Qual. Health Care 2006;18:220-3.

(253) Wong DR, Vander Salm TJ, Ali IS, Agnihotri AK, Bohmer RMJ, Torchiana DF. Prospective assessment of intraoperative precursor events during cardiac surgery.. Eur. J. Cardiothorac. Surg. 2006;29:447-55.

(254) Ochroch EA, Russell MW, Hanson WCIII, Devine GA, Cucchiara AJ, Weiner MG, Schwartz, SJ. The impact of continuous pulse oximetry monitoring on intensive care unit admissions from a postsurgical care floor. Anesth. Analg. 2006;102:868-75.

(255) McBride SC, Chiang VW, Goldmann DA, Landrigan CP. Preventable adverse events in infants hospitalized with bronchiolitis. Pediatrics 2005;116:603-8.

(256) Weingart SN. Beyond Babel: prospects for a universal patient safety taxonomy. Int. J. Qual. Health Care 2005;17:93-4.

(257) Weissman JS, Annas CL, Epstein AM, Schneider EC, Clarridge B, Kirle L, et al. Error reporting and disclosure systems: Views from hospital leaders. JAMA 2005;293:1359-66.

(258) Sundt TM, Brown JP, Uhlig PN, STS workforce on patient advocacy, communications. Focus on patient safety: Good news for the practicing surgeon. Ann. Thorac. Surg. 2005;79:11-5.

(259) Lim JK, Golub RM. Graduate medical education research in the 21st Century and JAMA on call. JAMA 2004;292:2913-5.

(260) Woolf SH, Kuzel AJ, Dovey SM, Phillips RLJr. A string of mistakes: The importance of cascade analysis in describing, counting, and preventing medical errors. Ann. Fam. Med. 2004;2:317-26.

(261) Clark PA. Medication errors in family practice, in hospitals and after discharge from the hospital. An ethical analysis. J. Law Med. Ethics 2004;32:349-57.

(262) Kohatsu ND, Gould D, Ross LK, Fox PJ. Characteristics associated with physician discipline: A case-control study. Arch. Intern. Med. 2004;164:653-8.

(263) Berger RG. Kichak JP. Computerized physician order entry: Helpful or harmful?. J. Am. Med. Inform. Assoc. 2004;11:100-3.

(264) Woolf SH. Patient safety is not enough: Targeting quality improvements to optimize the health of the population. Ann. Intern. Med. 2004;140:33-6.

(265) Margo CE. A pilot study in ophthalmology of inter-rater reliability in classifying diagnostic errors: an underinvestigated area of medical error. Qual. Saf. Health Care 2003;12:416-20.

(266) Curry JP, Hanson CWIII, Russell MW, Hanna C, Devine G, Ochroch EA. The use and effectiveness of electrocardiographic telemetry monitoring in a community hospital general care setting. Anesth. Analg. 2003;97:1483-7.

(267) Weingart SN, Iezzoni LI. Looking for medical injuries where the light is bright. JAMA 2003;290:1917-9.

(268) Kuzel AJ, Woolf SH, Engel JD, Gilchrist VJ, Frankel RM, LaVeist TA, Vincent C. Making the case for a qualitative study of medical errors in primary care. Qual. Health Res. 2003;13:743-80.

(269) Sage WM. Medical liability and patient safety. Health Aff. (Millwood) 2003;22:26-36.

(270) Fortescue EB, Kaushal R, Landrigan CP, McKenna KJ, Clapp MD, Federico F, et al. Prioritizing strategies for preventing medication errors and adverse drug events in pediatric inpatients. Pediatrics 2003;111:722-9.

(271) Lamb RM, Studdert DM, Bohmer RMJ, Berwick DM, Brennan TA. Hospital disclosure practices: Results of a national survey. Health Aff. (Millwood) 2003;22:73-83.

(272) Burke JP. Commentary. Qual. Saf. Health Care 2003;12:63-4.

(273) Ferraris VA, Ferraris SP. Risk stratification and comorbidity. Card. Surg. Adult 2003;2:187-224.

(274) Blendon RJ, DesRoches CM, Brodie M, Benson JM, Rosen AB, Schneider E, et al. Views of practicing physicians and the public on medical errors. New Engl. J. Med. 2002;347:1933-40.

(275) Lee TH. A broader concept of medicaleErrors. Engl. J. Med. 2002;347:1965-7.

(276) Freedman JE, Becker RC, Adams JE, Borzak S, Jesse RL, Newby LK, et al. Medication errors in acute cardiac care: An American Heart Association scientific statement from the Council on Clinical Cardiology Subcommittee on Acute Cardiac Care, Council on Cardiopulmonary and Critical Care, Council on Cardiovascular Nursing, and Council on Stroke. Circulation 2002;106:2623-9.

(277) Robinson AR, Hohmann KB, Rifkin JI, Topp D, Gilroy CM, Pickard JA, Anderson RJ. Physician and public opinions on quality of health care and the problem of medical errors. Arch. Intern. Med. 2002;162:2186-90.

(278) Hofer TP, Hayward RA. Are bad outcomes from questionable clinical decisions preventable medical errors? A case of cascade iatrogenesis. Ann. Intern. Med. 2002;137:327-33.

(279) Kaushal R, Bates DW. Information technology and medication safety: what is the benefit?. Qual. Saf. Health Care 2002;11:261-5.

(280) Kable AK, Gibberd RW, Spigelman AD. Adverse events in surgical patients in Australia. Int. J. Qual. Health Care 2002;14:269-76.

(281) Hickson GB, Federspiel CF, Pichert JW, Miller CS, Gauld-Jaeger J, Bost P. Patient complaints and malpractice risk. JAMA 2002;287:2951-7.

(282) Kloth DD. Prevention of chemotherapy medication errors. J. Pharmacy Pract. 2002;15:17-31.

(283) Eggimann P, Pittet D. Infection control in the ICU. Chest 2001;120:2059-93.

(284) Bunker JP. The role of medical care in contributing to health improvements within societies. Int. J. Epidemiol. 2001;30:1260-3.

(285) Sage WM. The lawyerization of medicine. J. Health Politics Policy Law 2001;26:1179-96.

(286) Kaushal R, Barker KN, Bates DW. How can information technology improve patient safety and reduce medication errors in children's health care? Arch. Pediatr. Adolesc. Med. 2001;155:1002-7.

(287) Hayward RA, Hofer TP. Estimating hospital deaths due to medical errors: Preventability is in the eye of the reviewer. JAMA 2001;286:415-20.

(288) Kaushal R, Bates DW, Landrigan C, McKenna KJ, Clapp MD, Federico F, Goldmann DA. Medication errors and adverse drug events in pediatric inpatients. JAMA 2001;285:2114-20.

(289) Hebert PC, Levin AV, Robertson G. Bioethics for clinicians: Disclosure of medical error. Can. Med. Assoc. J. 2001;164:509-13.

(290) Berlin L. Defending the "missed" radiographic diagnosis. Am. J. Roentgenol. 2001;176:317-22.

(291) Hughes CM, Honig P, Phillips J, Woodcock J, Anderson RE, McDonald CJ, et al. How many deaths are due to medical errors? JAMA 2000;284:2187.

(292) Richardson WC, Berwick DM, Bisgard JC, Newhall C, Melker RJ, Brennan TA. The Institute of Medicine report on medical errors. New Engl. J. Med. 2000;343:663-5.

(293) Kakaiya R, Migden D, Van Oeveren EL, Mohr JC, Gostin LO. The past and future of medical malpractice litigation. JAMA 2000;284:827-9.

(294) McDonald CJ, Weiner M, Hui SL. Deaths due to medical errors are exaggerated in Institute of Medicine Report. JAMA 2000;284:93-5.

(295) Grof C, Grof S. Spiritual emergency: The understanding and treatment of transpersonal crises. ReVISION 1986;8(2):7-20.

(296) Grof S. Psychodynamic factors in depression and psychosis: Observations from modern consciousness research. New York: New York University Press, 1987.

(297) Grof S. The cosmic game: Explorations of the frontiers of human consciousness. SUNY Series in Transpersonal and Humanistic Psychology. State University of New York Press, New York, 1998.

(298) Grof C, Grof S, Feuerstein G, Wilber K. Problems on the path: Clinical concerns. New York: Perigee Books, 1993.

(299) Schopenhauer A. Die Welt als Wille und Vorstellung (The World as Will and Representation) [third edition, two volumes] Leipzig: FA Brockhaus, 1859.

(300) Bø K, Berghmans B, Mørkved S, Van Kampen M. Evidence-based physical physical therapy for the pelvic floor. Bridging science and clinical practice. New York: Elsevier Butterworth Heinemann, 2007.

(301) Leichsenring F, Leibing E. Psychodynamic psychotherapy: a systematic review of techniques, indications and empirical evidence. Psychol. Psychother. 2007;80(Pt 2):217-28.

(302) Leichsenring F, Rabung S, Leibing E. The efficacy of short-term psychodynamic psychotherapy in specific psychiatric disorders: a meta-analysis. Arch. Gen. Psychiatry 2004;61(12):1208-16.

(303) Leichsenring F. Are psychodynamic and psychoanalytic therapies effective?: A review of empirical data. Int. J. Psychoanal. 2005;86(Pt 3):841-68.

(304) Shek DT, Ma HK.Design of a positive youth development program in Hong Kong. Int. J. Adolesc. Med. Health 2006;18(3):315-27.

(305) Gøtzche PC. Reference bias in reports of drug trials. BMJ 1987;295;654-6.

(306) van Tulder M, Furlan A, Bombardier C, Bouter L; Editorial Board of the Cochrane Collaboration Back Review Group. Updated method guidelines for systematic reviews in the Cochrane Collaboration back review group. Spine 2003;28(12):1290-9.

(307) Higgins J, Green S. Cochrane handbook for systematic reviews of interventions version 5.0.0. edn. Oxford: Cochrane Collaboration, 2008.
(308) Moher D, Cook DJ, Eastwood S, Olkin I, Rennie D, Stroup DF. Improving the quality of reports of meta-analyses of randomized controlled trials: the QUOROM statement. Quality of Reporting of Meta-analyses. Lancet 1999;354:1896-900.
(309) Blaylock R. Swine Flu: Massive Conspiracy-Cover-Up. http://www.conspiracyplanet.com/channel.cfm?channelid=47 andcontentid=6421andpage=2 Accessed 2009-12-15.
(310) Halla J. Drug related hospital admission in subspecialties of internal medicine. Dan. Med. Bull. 1996; 45(2):141-55.
(311) Ventegodt S, Merrick J. Principles of holistic psychiatry. A textbook of holistic medicine for mental disorders. New York: Nova Science, 2011.
(312) Ventegodt S, Merrick J. Sexology from a holistic point of view. A textbook of classical and modern sexology. New York: Nova Science, 2011.
(313) Andersen NV. Pharmaceutical companies puts illegal TV-commercials. Every second "information campaign" from pharmaceutical companies are Illegal concludes the Radio- and TV court." [Medicinvirksomheder sender ulovlige tv-reklamer. Hver anden "oplysningskampagne" fra lægemiddelvirksomheder på tv er ulovlige, fastslår Radio og TV-Nævnet.] Ugeskr Læger 2009;171 (21):1737.
(314) "Pharmaindustrie: Mehr Geld für Werbung als für Forschung - Nachrichten Wissenschaft - WELT ONLINE" [in German]. Welt.de. 2008-01-04. http://www.welt.de/wissenschaft/article1510150/Mehr_Geld_fuer_Werbung_als_fuer_Forschung.html. Retrieved 2009-04-20.
(315) Ventegodt S, Merrick J. A review of the Danish National Drug Directory: Who provides the data for the register? Int. J. Adolesc. Med. Health 2010;22(2):197-212.
(316) www.medicine.dk accessed 2009-12-16.
(317) Christensen PM, Kristiansen IS. Number-Needed-to-treat (NNT): Needs treatment with care. Basic Clin. Pharmacolol. Toxicol. 2006; 99 (1) :12-16.
(318) Halvorsen PA, Kristiansen IS, Aasland AND et al. Medical doctors perception of the "number needed to treat (NNT). A survey of doctors recommendation for two therapies with different NNT. Scand. J. Prim. Health Care 2003; 21 (3) :162-6.
(319) Ventegodt S, Merrick J, Andersen NJ. Quality of life as medicine: A pilot study of patients with chronic ilness and pain. Scientific World Journal 2003;3:520-32.
(320) Ventegodt S, Merrick J, Andersen NJ. Quality of life as medicine II: A pilot study of a five-day "quality of life and health" cure for patients with alcoholism. Scientific World Journal 2003;3:842-52.
(321) Ventegodt S, Clausen B, Langhorn M, Kromann M, Andersen NJ, Merrick J. Quality of life as medicine III. A qualitative analysis of the effect of a five day intervention with existential holistic group therapy or a quality of life course as a modern rite of passage. Scientific World Journal 2004;4:124-33.
(322) Beck RT. Ventegodt: "Jeg er tilbage på banen". Copenhagen: Politiken, 2006 Jan 20.
(323) www.inter-uni.net.
(324) www.bolenreport.net/feature_articles Accessed 2008-11-04.
(325) Film director Peter Engberg, Personal communication, 2009.

INDEX

A

B

D

E

F

G

H

I

J

K

L

M

N

O

P

Q

R

S